W9-BCN-638

Techniques in the Clinical Supervision of Teachers

Techniques in the Clinical Supervision of Teachers

Preservice and Inservice Applications

Keith A. Acheson

Meredith Damien Gall

University of Oregon

LONGMAN/New York and London

TECHNIQUES IN THE CLINICAL SUPERVISION OF TEACHERS
Preservice and Inservice Applications

Longman Inc., New York
Associated companies, branches, and representatives
throughout the world.

Sponsoring Editor: Nicole Benevento
Production Editor: Elinor Weinberger
Interior Design: Pencils Portfolio, Inc.
Cover Design: Edgar Blakeney
Manufacturing and Production Supervisor: Kris Becker
Composition: A&S Graphics, Inc.
Printing and Binding: Fairfield Graphics

Manufactured in the United States of America

Printing: 10 9 8 7
Year: 9 8 7 6 5

Library of Congress Cataloging in Publication Data

Acheson, Keith A   1925–
  Techniques in the Clinical supervision of teachers.

  Includes index.
  1. Teaching. 2. Classroom management. 3. Audio-
visual equipment. I. Gall, Meredith D., 1942–
joint author. II. Title.
LB1025.2.A216   317.1'02   79-17087
ISBN 0-582-28122-9
ISBN 0-582-28121-0 pbk.

Contents

Acknowledgments

Some of the ideas in this book were developed at Stanford University in the early 1960s along with techniques for using videotape and other forms of feedback in the training of preservice and inservice teachers. People in that project who influenced the ideas, research, and applications were Robert Bush, Dwight Allen, Fred McDonald, Norman Boyan, Horace Aubertine, Bill Johnson, Jim Olivero, Frank McGraw, Al Robertson and Jimmy Fortune.

Both authors, along with John Hansen, worked on earlier versions of the techniques presented in the book as part of a project sponsored by the Far West Laboratory for Educational Research and Development. The support and suggestions of Walter Borg and Ned Flanders were especially helpful. The materials that grew out of the project were used in many workshops and were published by the Association of California School Administrators and later at Florida State University. Ed Beaubier and Art Thayer were instrumental during this phase of the materials' development, as was Ray Hull.

For the past decade, research conducted at the University of Oregon by the authors, their colleagues, and students has influenced the attitudes and recommendations reflected in the book. We thank Peter Titze, Wes Tolliver, Michael Carl, Colin Yarham, Gary Martin, Jim Shinn, Judy Aubrecht, John Suttle, and Kathy Lovell. Also, several professional associations and state education departments have supported the development and dissemination of the ideas and procedures recounted herein. We are especially grateful to the Confederation of Oregon School Administrators and Ozzie Rose, the Oregon State Department of Education and Ron Burge, the Nevada Association of School Administrators, the principals' and superintendents' associations in Washington and British Columbia, the Nebraska Association for Supervision and Curriculum Development, the British Columbia Ministry of Education and Russ Leskiw, the National Academy of School Executives, and the many school districts that have conducted workshops and conferences using our materials and personnel.

The research of Dale Bolton at the University of Washington and Rob Spaulding at San Jose State has influenced our conclusions. Reports of our work have been presented at two conventions of the American Educational Research Association, once in a paper written in collaboration with Paul Tucker and Cal Zigler and more recently in a symposium with members of the Teacher Corps Research Adaptation Cluster. We also thank the administrators and teachers who reacted to earlier drafts of the materials in three annual workshops conducted on Orcas Island in Washington State.

A Note to the Instructor

The content of this book can be taught in several formats. We recommend taking up observation techniques first, giving the participants opportunities to practice in a live setting whenever possible and to share experiences and data with other members of the class. Planning conferences can be introduced as a topic while students are still trying out different observation systems. An analysis of a planning conference makes a reasonable assignment. After feedback conferences have been discussed, students should have the chance to work through at least one complete cycle with a teacher. Teachers should be selected for their willingness to let the observers practice their skills. Observers who have student teachers assigned to them, and principals who have a faculty to work with, should have no difficulty finding opportunities to apply their new skills.

Simulated situations can be set up to allow participants to practice observing short lessons taught by classmates to their peers. Participants can also practice conference skills in role-playing sessions with classmates, using data supplied by the instructor; an observer for each pair of role players allows for subsequent debriefing and discussion. Tape recordings of conferences are useful in the analysis process, but we find that many teachers are reluctant to permit tape recording unless they understand clearly what use will be made of the tapes and that they will not be evaluated or embarrassed in the process.

A number of activities, exercises, and assignments can be used in conjunction with the printed materials and instructor presentations. Listing what class members feel are the crucial competencies of teaching will stimulate interest in the aspects of teaching effectiveness discussed in chapter 2.

Tape recordings of classroom interaction can be used to practice writing selected verbatim comments, questions, or responses. Films or videotapes showing nonverbal behaviors also can be useful. A prepared tape (or psychodrama) of a conference gives class members something tangible to react to when studying conference techniques. Overhead projector transparencies of data from seating charts or other observation instruments can serve as a focus for analysis and discussion.

Teaching the skills for coding interaction requires some structured practice. We suggest having a tape recording that has been carefully coded by an expert so that class members can be given feedback when they practice.

Instructor presentations on topics such as research on teaching or supervision can augment the material on these topics in the book. Small-group discussions in which participants share their experiences, data, and opinions have been valuable activities in our courses.

A Note to the Reader

This book is about the clinical supervision of teachers. Several texts on clinical supervision have been published in the last decade, but in general they have emphasized theory and research on clinical supervision. Our book is practical in intent. We emphasize the techniques of clinical supervision, the "nuts and bolts" of how to work with teachers to help them improve their classroom teaching.

In preparing the text, we were guided by a set of objectives to help you, the supervisor, develop

- An understanding of the three phases of clinical supervision: planning conference, classroom observation, and feedback conference;
- Knowledge and skill in using specific techniques in conferences with teachers and in observing their classroom teaching;
- Understanding of issues and problems in doing clinical supervision;
- Understanding of role differences of the supervisor as facilitator, evaluator, counselor, and curriculum adviser;
- A positive attitude toward clinical supervision as a method of promoting teacher growth.

The textbook format is better suited for helping you achieve knowledge and understanding objectives than it is for helping you achieve skill-related objectives. If you are typical of most educators, you did not learn how to teach by reading textbooks. You learned how to teach by practicing the act of teaching in actual classroom situations. (We hope you had a skillful supervisor to assist you!) Textbooks may have facilitated this process by suggesting specific techniques for you to try.

The same principle applies to acquiring skill as a clinical supervisor. We would like to think that this textbook is sufficient to train you to be a highly skilled supervisor. Our experience suggests otherwise. You will need to practice and receive feedback on each conference and observation technique if you are to incorporate them into your supervisory repertoire. It would help, too, if you have the opportunity to observe supervisors who can model these techniques.

Building principals, school district personnel, and teacher educators in colleges and universities may be required to do teacher supervision as part of their duties. These professional educators need to be skilled in the processes of clinical teacher supervision. If you currently supervise teachers or if you plan to do so in the future, this book was written with you in mind.

The book is organized into four units. The first unit provides necessary background for understanding techniques of clinical supervision. The next two units describe specific techniques for conducting clinical conferences and collecting observation data. The final unit presents case studies and answers questions frequently asked about clinical supervision.

List of Clinical Supervision Techniques

Some readers are helped by seeing all the clinical supervision techniques in a single list. Here is a list of the techniques presented in this book. Each technique is keyed to the pages on which it is discussed.

First Phase: Planning Conference
1. Identify the teacher's concerns about instruction (pages 44–46).
2. Translate the teacher's concerns into observable behavior (pages 46–49).
3. Identify procedures for improving the teacher's instruction (pages 49–51).
4. Assist the teacher in setting self-improvement goals (pages 51–52).
5. Arrange a time for classroom observation (pages 52–53).
6. Select an observation instrument and behaviors to be recorded (pages 53–54).
7. Clarify the instructional context in which data will be recorded (pages 54–55).

Second Phase: Classroom Observation
    Selective Verbatim:
8. Teacher questions (pages 90–95).
9. Teacher feedback. (pages 95–100).
10. Teacher directions and structuring statements (pages 100–102).
    Seating Chart Observational Records:
11. At task (pages 105–13).
12. Verbal flow (pages 113–19).
13. Movement patterns (pages 119–25).

    Wide Lens Techniques:
14. Anecdotal records (pages 127–31).
15. Video and audio recordings (pages 131–34).

Unit I

Introduction to Clinical Supervision

Overview

Clinical supervision has as its goal the professional development of teachers, with an emphasis on improving teachers' classroom performance. Chapter 1 introduces you to the basic characteristics of clinical supervision and compares it with other forms of teacher supervision. As the goal of clinical supervision is effective teaching, chapter 2 presents criteria of effective teaching proposed by educators and teachers. Supervisor and teacher can use these criteria to define for themselves what is meant by "effective teaching."

Objectives

The purpose of this unit is to help you develop:

Understanding of the basic processes and goals of clinical supervision.

Understanding of why teachers traditionally have had negative attitudes toward supervision.

Understanding of how clinical supervision differs from other forms of teacher supervision.

Understanding of the relationship between clinical supervision and teacher evaluation.

Knowledge about the current state of research on clinical supervision's effectiveness.

1

Understanding of different perspectives from which to define effective teaching.

Knowledge about criteria of effective teaching that have been discovered through research.

Skill in defining what is meant by effective teaching.

1

The Nature of Clinical Supervision

An Example

"What gripes me about this so-called supervision is that the principal only comes into my classroom once a year for about an hour. It's a scary, unpleasant experience. I wouldn't mind if I was being supervised by someone who's been a success in the classroom; but usually it's someone who was a poor teacher who's been pushed into an administrative position; and, to top it off, that person usually has had no training whatsoever in how to supervise."—From a conversation with a sixth-grade teacher

The spirit of clinical supervision is difficult to capture in words. Clinical supervision is a process, a distinctive style of relating to teachers. For this process to be effective, the clinical supervisor's mind, emotions, and actions must work together to achieve the primary goal of clinical supervision: the professional development of the preservice or inservice teacher.

Although we acknowledge the unitary nature of clinical supervision, our book is primarily analytical. It attempts to tease out and describe the components and techiques of clinical supervision. This analytical approach is useful as an instructional device, but it does not allow you to view clinical supervision as a whole. As a way of dealing with this problem, we present an episode from an actual case of clinical supervision.

3

Arthur Harris, a university supervisor, was assigned to supervise Jim, a student teacher at a local junior high school. Harris had an initial meeting with Jim to get acquainted, discuss the supervisory role, and answer questions. He then met with the two teachers in whose classrooms Jim would work and with the school's principal. The two teachers gave Jim several weeks to observe their classes, become acquainted with the students, and prepare several social studies units.

Arthur Harris viewed his initial role as providing support and encouragement to Jim. Once Jim had found his bearings, Harris explained the procedures of clinical supervision and initiated a supervisory cycle by asking Jim to state his lesson plan for the class on Africa that Harris would observe later in the week. Jim's plan was to organize the students into three groups and have each group read a different article about Rhodesia. Then Jim wanted students in each group to state what they learned from the articles and answer questions about them.

Supervisor Harris and Jim agreed that it would be helpful to collect data on verbal interaction patterns in the lesson. Two specific areas of focus were selected: (1) Jim's responses to students' answers and ideas, which Harris would record using selective verbatim (technique 9); and (2) the distribution of student talk during the lesson, which would be recorded on a seating chart (technique 12).

Exhibit 1.1 shows a sample of the data collected by Arthur Harris using each technique. When Jim and Harris met the following week for a feedback conference, Jim was able to use the data to reach his own conclusions about how the lesson went. Supervisor Harris initiated this process by asking, "What do these data tell you about your teaching?" (technique 23). Jim realized that he had not praised or elaborated on student ideas other than simply to acknowledge them. Also, Jim saw that he was successful in getting students to talk, but the distribution of talk was unbalanced: students nearest the teacher, and one student in particular, did most of the speaking.

Arthur Harris's next move in the feedback conference was to ask Jim how he would explain why these verbal patterns occurred (technique 24). Jim commented that he had heard in his methods courses about the importance of responding constructively to student ideas, but he had not made the connection to his own teaching behavior until now. As for the distribution of student talk, Jim stated he was simply unaware that the imbalance had occurred. He realized, though, that he probably called a number of times on the student who talked the most because he could depend on her to give good answers.

T: Do u know what was being discussed in this article?

S: No.

T: Well, in 1964 ... backfire from all this ... Do u understand what that will mean?

S: ——

S: ——

T: That's true. OK. We know Russia is 1 of leading producers of chromium. What do we use chromium for?

S: Automobiles.

S: Makes things shine.

T: OK. Russia ... What wld that mean?

S: We'd be ...

T: OK.

S: And they'd use that against us.

T: Another thing in the article that was important?

S: Blacks can vote ... Not many do.

T: Not many do. Do you get feeling for how blacks in Rhodesia ...

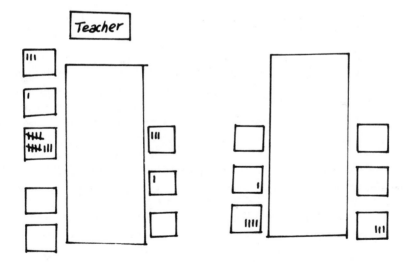

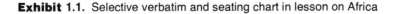

Exhibit 1.1. Selective verbatim and seating chart in lesson on Africa

Supervisor Harris asked Jim what he might do based on these observations (technique 25). Jim said he would practice using praise in his next lessons and would make an effort to call on more students. Harris suggested several ways that Jim might acknowledge student ideas and incorporate them in the lesson. He also suggested that a different arrangement of desks—perhaps a semicircle or circle—might encourage students to express more ideas and engage in discussion among themselves.

This brief example illustrates the three phases of the clinical supervision cycle: planning conference, classroom observation, and feedback conference. The example also makes clear that clinical supervision focuses on the teacher's actual classroom performance and includes the teacher as an active participant in the supervisory process.

The "Problem" of Teacher Supervision

Most teachers do not like to be supervised, even though it is a required part of their training and professional work. They react defensively to supervision, and they do not find it helpful.

This generalization undoubtedly has exceptions. Some teachers profit from supervision, and some gifted supervisors are popular and effective in working with teachers. Yet the weight of evidence supports the generalization. In a study of 2500 teachers, Wiles found that only a small fraction of them (1.5 percent) perceived their supervisor as a source of new ideas.[1] Cogan conducted several studies of teacher supervision, on the basis of which he concluded that "psychologically [supervision] is almost inevitably viewed as an active threat to the teacher, possibly endangering his professional standing and undermining his confidence."[2] More recently, Blumberg reviewed studies of teacher supervision conducted by himself and others and found that teachers view supervision "as a part of the system that exists but that does not play an important role in their professional lives, almost like an organizational ritual that is no longer relevant."[3]

The prevalence of teacher hostility to supervision would suggest that schools abandon it entirely. A more hopeful conclusion is that teachers are hostile, not to supervision, but to the style of supervision they typically receive. *Teachers might react positively to a supervisory style that is more responsive to their concerns and aspirations.* Clinical supervision is based on this premise.

Before describing what clinical supervision is, let us examine some supervisory practices to which teachers react negatively. In traditional inservice supervision, the supervisor—usually the school principal—initiates the supervisory process to evaluate the teacher's performance. The evaluation function may be mandated by state law, as in California and Oregon, or by the local school board.

This situation creates two problems at the start. First, supervision becomes equated with evaluation. People tend to be anxious when they know they are being evaluated, especially if negative evaluations threaten their jobs. No wonder, then, that teachers react negatively to supervision. The second problem is that supervision arises from a need the supervisor has, rather than from a felt need of the teacher.

Because traditional supervision tends to be unpleasant, interaction between supervisor and teacher is avoided or minimized. Unfortunately, this practice compounds the problem. The supervisor may show up unannounced at the teacher's classroom to observe what is happening. The teacher has no knowledge of what the supervisor might observe and evaluate. Is the supervisor interested in the neatness of the classroom, in the students' apparent interest in their work, in the objectives and teaching strategy of the lesson, or perhaps in the degree to which classroom control is maintained? The supervisor, on the other hand, may not have planned what to observe and evaluate. The result is that classroom visitation data are likely to be unsystematic, highly subjective, and vague.

The follow-up to classroom visitation is not likely to improve matters. Typically the supervisor completes a rating checklist and writes an evaluative report on the teacher's performance. The teacher may not have an opportunity to confer with the supervisor about the observational data and evaluative criteria used in the report, even though the report may be used in important decisions relating to the teacher's promotion and tenure.

This highly directive form of supervision reflects the historical role of supervisors as school "inspectors." As far back as the early eighteenth century, lay committees in Boston were charged with inspecting schools periodically. The purpose of inspection was to determine whether instructional standards were being maintained. School inspection by lay committees continued until schools grew large enough to require more than one teacher in each school. The inspection function then became the responsibility of one of the teachers, who was known as the "principal teacher." Eventually the title was shortened to "principal." Although other models of supervision have been advocated in recent years, many principals probably still perceive their supervisory role as that of inspector.

Clinical Supervision—A Definition

The preceding description of teacher supervision is overdrawn, yet it characterizes what some supervisors do some of the time. To the extent that the portrayal is accurate, it accounts for teachers' pervasive negative feelings about supervision. We wish to promote an alternative model of supervision that is interactive rather than directive, democratic rather than authoritarian, teacher-centered rather than supervisor-centered. This supervisory style is called clinical supervision.

We use the label *clinical supervision* because the model presented here is based directly on the methods developed by Morris Cogan, Robert Goldhammer, and others at the Harvard School of Education in the 1960s.[4] "Clinical" is meant to suggest a face-to-face relationship between teacher and supervisor and a focus on the teacher's actual behavior in the classroom. As Goldhammer puts it, "Given close observation, detailed observational data, face-to-face interaction between the supervisor and teacher, and an intensity of focus that binds the two together in an intimate professional relationship, the meaning of 'clinical' is pretty well filled out."[5]

The word "clinical" can also connote pathology, a connotation that should not be applied to the model of teacher supervision presented here. We certainly do not wish you to think that clinical supervision is always a "remedy" applied by the supervisor to deficient or unhealthy behavior exhibited by the teacher. To avoid this implied meaning of clinical supervision, we considered using the term *teacher-centered supervision*. One nice feature of this label is that it parallels the method of "person-centered counseling" popularized by Carl Rogers,[6] with which clinical supervision has much in common. Nevertheless, we settled on "clinical supervision" as more descriptive because it continues the usage of the group at Harvard who originated this model of supervision.

Clinical supervision acknowledges the need for teacher evaluation, under the condition that the teacher participates with the supervisor in this process. The primary emphasis of clinical supervision is on professional development, however. *It is supervision to help the teacher improve his or her instructional performance.*

How is this goal to be accomplished? The supervisor begins the process of supervision by holding a conference with the teacher. In the conference the teacher has an opportunity to state personal concerns, needs, and aspirations. The supervisor's role is to help the teacher clarify these perceptions so that the two of them have a clear picture of the teacher's current instruction, the teacher's view of ideal instruction, and whether there is a discrepancy between the two. Next, supervisor and teacher explore new techniques that the teacher might try in order to move the instruction toward the ideal.

This first phase of supervision, done properly, can be helpful to the teacher. Teaching is a lonely profession. Most teachers (i.e., those who do not work in a team teaching context) are deprived of access to colleagues with whom they can share perceptions. Supervision can satisfy this important need of teachers.

The planning conference also provides teachers with an opportunity to reflect on their teaching. Many teachers have a vague anxiety about the effectiveness of their teaching. They do not know whether they are doing a good job, whether a "problem" student can be helped, whether their instruction can be improved. Teachers rarely have the opportunity to observe other teachers' classroom performance, which might provide a basis for reflecting on their own performance. Supervisors can meet this need by using a different approach—helping the teacher clarify goals, collecting observational data on classroom events, and analyzing the data for discrepancies. For teachers who are not aware of their goals or how they "come across" in the classroom, this process can be a useful guide.

The planning conference often results in a cooperative decision by teacher and supervisor to collect observational data. For example, a teacher we know had a vaguely defined concern that he was turning off the brighter students in the class. In the planning conference the teacher developed the hypothesis that perhaps he was spending the majority of his time with the slower students in the class and ignoring the needs of the brighter students. Together, teacher and supervisor decided that it might be helpful to do a verbal flow analysis (technique 6) of the teacher's discussion behavior. This analysis involves observation of the students with whom the teacher initiates interaction and how he responds to each student's ideas. The teacher and the supervisor also decided it would be worthwhile for the teacher to collect class assignments over a two-week period to determine their level of difficulty and challenge.

It is curious how rarely we collect data on different aspects of the teacher's classroom performance. In the field of sports, for example, the athlete watches closely the statistical data that summarize observations of his performance—number of home runs in baseball, percentage of completed passes in football, final and intermediate times in track events, and so forth. Also, the athlete is exposed constantly to videotape replays of his performance so that he can perfect his technique. In professions such as medicine, business, and law, the practitioner has access to a number of indicators that directly

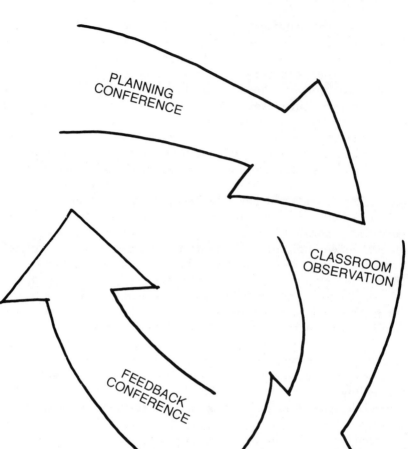

Figure 1.1. The three phases of the clinical supervision cycle

reflect quality of performance—number of lives saved, salary based on fees, sales figures. Additionally, practitioners often hear expressions of satisfaction or dissatisfaction from their clients. *We need to provide teachers with similar indicators of performance, based on direct or indirect observation.*

The final phase of clinical supervision is for teacher and supervisor to participate in a feedback conference. Together they review the observational data, with the supervisor encouraging the teacher to make his or her own inferences about teaching effectiveness. For example, in viewing a videotape of their performance, teachers usually notice a number of areas in which they need to improve. They comment that they hadn't known how much they talk in class, that they tend to ignore or fail to acknowledge student comments, that they do not speak forcefully enough, and the like.

As the teacher reviews the observational data, the feedback conference often turns into a planning conference—with teacher and supervisor deciding cooperatively to collect further observational data or plan a self-improvement program.

In brief, clinical supervision is a model of supervision that contains three phases: planning conference, classroom observation, and feedback conference. The model is shown graphically in figure 1.1. The most distinctive features of clinical supervision are its emphases on direct teacher-supervisor interaction and the teacher's professional development.

Richard Weller has offered a formal definition of clinical supervision: "Clinical supervision may be defined as supervision focused upon the improvement of instruction by means of systematic cycles of planning, observation, and intensive intellectual analysis of actual teaching performances in the interest of rational modification."[7] In addition to providing this succinct but accurate definition, Weller isolated the essential characteristics and assumptions of clinical supervision as described in the literature. This list of characteristics and assumptions is presented below. The characteristics are operationalized in the set of conference and observation techniques presented in chapters 3 through 9.

Essential Characteristics and Assumptions of Clinical Supervision[8]

1. The improvement of instruction requires that teachers learn specific intellectual and behavioral skills.
2. The primary function of the supervisor is to teach these skills to the teacher:
   a. Skills of complex analytic perception of the instructional process;
   b. Skills of rational analysis of the instructional process based on explicit observational evidence;
   c. Skills of curriculum innovation, implementation, and experimentation;
   d. Skills of teaching performance.

3. The supervisory focus is on what and how teachers teach; its main objective is to improve instruction, not change the teacher's personality.

4. The supervisory focus in planning and analysis is best anchored in the making and testing of instructional hypotheses based on observational evidence.

5. The supervisory focus is on instructional issues that are small in number, educationally vital, intellectually accessible to the teacher, and amenable to change.

6. The supervisory focus is on constructive analysis and the reinforcement of successful patterns rather than on the condemnation of unsuccessful patterns.

7. The supervisory focus is based on observational evidence, not on unsubstantiated value judgments.

8. The cycle of planning, teaching, and analysis is a continuing one that builds upon past experience.

9. Supervision is a dynamic process of give-and-take in which supervisors and interns are colleagues in search of mutual educational understanding.

10. The supervisory process is primarily one of verbal interaction centered on the analysis of instruction.

11. The individual teacher has both the freedom and the responsibility to initiate issues, analyze and improve his own teaching, and develop a personal teaching style.

12. Supervision is itself patterned and amenable to comparable processes of complex perception, rational analysis, and improvement.

13. The supervisor has both the freedom and the responsibility to analyze and evaluate his own supervision in a manner similar to a teacher's analysis and evaluation of his instruction.

The Goals of Clinical Supervision

Planning conferences, classroom observation, and feedback conferences are the major activities of clinical supervision. *The major aim of these activities is the improvement of teachers' classroom instruction.* In this respect clinical supervision is a key technique for promoting the professional development of teachers.

The aim of clinical supervision can be analyzed into more specific goals as follows:

(1) *To provide teachers with objective feedback on the current state of their instruction.* Clinical supervision, in its most basic form, holds up a

mirror so that teachers can see what they are actually doing while teaching. What teachers do may be quite different from what teachers think they are doing. For example, many teachers believe they are good at encouraging students to express their ideas *until* they listen to an audiotape of their lessons. Then teachers discover the extent to which they dominate the lesson; typically, two thirds of classroom talk is by the teacher. Receiving objective feedback often is sufficient stimulus for teachers to initiate a self-improvement process.

(1) *To diagnose and solve instructional problems.* Clinical supervisors use conference techniques and observational records to help teachers pinpoint specific discrepancies between what they are doing and what they ought to do. At times teachers are able to diagnose these discrepancies on their own. On other occasions the skilled intervention of a supervisor is necessary. A parallel situation exists in classroom instruction. Sometimes students can self-diagnose a problem they are having in learning, and they can take remedial steps on the basis of this information. At other times students are stymied by their inability to learn a particular subject, and the teacher is needed to diagnose and remediate.

(3) *To help teachers develop skill in using instructional strategies.* If clinical supervision's only purpose were to help the teacher solve immediate problems and crises, its value would be severely limited. The supervisor would be needed each time the teacher had a "brush fire" to be put out. This is not true. The skillful supervisor uses the clinical conference and observation data to help the teacher develop enduring patterns of behavior—what we call "instructional strategies." These strategies are effective in promoting learning, motivating students, and managing the classroom. The observational techniques presented in chapters 6–9 and the criteria for effective teaching in chapter 2 deal with instructional strategies most educators believe effective. Teachers can practice these strategies and can receive objective data on improvement resulting from practice.

(4) *To evaluate teachers for promotion, tenure, or other decisions.* This is the most controversial function of clinical supervision. Some supervisors avoid evaluation, but most supervisors are required by the school district or college of education to evaluate the teacher's competence, usually at the end of the supervisory cycle. Although clinical supervision emphasizes the teacher's professional development, the objective data collected through systematic classroom observation provide one basis for evaluating the teacher's competence. As we discuss later in the chapter, the "sting" of evaluation can be lessened if, as part of the clinical supervision process, the supervisor shares with the teacher the criteria and standards to be used in the evaluation report.

(5)   *To help teachers develop a positive attitude about continuous professional development*. A major goal of clinical supervision is to help the teacher realize that training does not end with the completion of certification requirements. Teachers need to view themselves as professionals, which means, in part, that they engage in self-development and skill training as a career-long effort. The clinical supervisor can model this aspect of professionalism by a willingness to develop new supervisory skills.

Other Types of Teacher Supervision

The purpose of *clinical* supervision can be further clarified by comparing it with other kinds of teacher supervision.

Counseling. Many teachers—especially student teachers and first-year teachers—have overt anxiety and insecurity about their ability to perform in the classroom. Also teachers may experience temporary crises in their personal lives that interfere with classroom performance. Some teachers may suffer from chronic emotional problems (e.g., depression or unprovoked outbursts of anger) that disrupt their teaching effectiveness.

Sensitive supervisors respond to teachers' anxiety and insecurity by providing emotional support and reassurance. They also may make an effort to deal with more serious problems or may refer a teacher to appropriate specialists. In carrying out these functions, the supervisor is performing the role of counselor. Clinical supervision may also incorporate these functions, but its focus is on the teacher's instructional performance rather than the teacher's personal problems.

Another problem that arises in teacher supervision centers on career decisions. Student teachers often wonder whether they are cut out to be teachers. They may ask for assistance in seeking a teaching position or for advice about additional education. Experienced teachers may feel undecided about whether to remain in the teaching profession, seek a transfer to another school, or teach a different content area and grade level. The supervisor who advises a teacher about such problems is performing a counseling function rather than a clinical supervision function.

Curriculum Support. Teachers sometimes ask their supervisors for advice about curriculum materials they are using. Are the materials suitable? How should they be used? Are alternative materials available? A teacher may have other curriculum concerns as well: the amount of time to spend on each curriculum topic, procedures for organizing a course of study, new curriculum policy and guidelines in the school district.

Supervision in the form of curriculum support can be very helpful to the teacher, but it should not be equated with clinical supervision. Clinical supervision focuses directly on *actual observable events of teaching*. In contrast, curriculum support focuses on materials, objectives, and philosophy of instruction. These are major influences on teaching, but they are not the teaching act itself.

A Note of Caution. Counseling and curriculum support are important, legitimate functions of teacher supervision. Teachers do experience emotional problems and curriculum concerns that may impede their instructional effectiveness. Nevertheless, a teacher may use these problems and concerns as an excuse to avoid dealing with difficulties in the act of teaching.

For example, a teacher may feel uncomfortable about the fact that students in his class are generally unruly. Yet he does not wish to confront this problem and does not want the supervisor to notice what is happening. Thus he steers the supervisory conference in the direction of problems and events that exist outside his classroom. (We know of instances where teacher and supervisor used their time together to talk about the problems of other teachers in the school.) When these situations occur, the clinical supervisor should listen sensitively to the teacher's comments but then tactfully steer the conference back to the teacher's own classroom behavior.

Teacher Evaluation and Clinical Supervision

Supervisors face a conflict caused by being caught between two roles—evaluator and facilitator. Supervisors often ask, "How can I help teachers grow as persons and as classroom instructors when they know that, eventually, I must make a written evaluation of their effectiveness?" So great is the conflict that some educators have argued for a separation in roles. Thus, some supervisors would evaluate teachers' performance in a manner similar to the traditional "inspector" role. Other supervisors would devote themselves to promoting teachers' development.

Teachers feel the conflict, too. They do not know whether to rely on the supervisor for support or avoid the supervisor for fear of being criticized.

This book is strongly oriented toward the role of clinical supervisor as facilitator, yet we acknowledge that most supervisors must also evaluate teachers. Preservice teachers are usually evaluated at the end of their student-teaching experience by the university supervisor and cooperating teachers. These evaluations are put in teachers' placement files and influence their chances of obtaining teaching positions. Evaluation reports of inservice teachers may influence salary increases, promotions, and tenure decisions.

We have no solution for the problem created by the supervisor's dual role of facilitator and evaluator. But the following observations may help you and the teachers you supervise work toward your own resolution of the problem.

The conflict between facilitation and evaluation is not unique to teacher supervision; supervisors in all occupations and professions face the same problem. Even teachers must play the dual role of evaluator and facilitator. Teachers are charged with the responsibility of helping their students learn, but they also are required to evaluate how well students have learned relative one to another.[9]

Remember that the "sting" of evaluation can be lessened by a skillful supervisor. Teachers are most threatened when they are unaware of the criteria by which they will be judged and when they do not trust the evaluator's ability to be fair. These concerns can be alleviated by involving the teacher in the evaluative process—for example, by sharing the evaluative criteria beforehand and by basing the evaluation on objective observational data shared with the teacher. This process of sharing ideally results in teacher and supervisor working together rather than at cross-purposes.

The experience of our colleagues in the teaching profession and our own experience indicates that the vast majority of teachers are effective and can improve with supervision and training. Less effective teachers usually self-select out of the profession either during the preservice phase or during the first few years in the field. The realization that probability is working for them (i.e., they are more likely to be evaluated positively than negatively) helps many teachers accept the evaluative function of supervision.

Finally, we remind you of the old truism that people often learn more from their failures than from their successes. Even a negative evaluation may provide a growth experience. Supervisor and teacher may find that a negative evaluation of the teacher's performance is painful for both of them, especially if it results in the teacher's leaving the profession. One can only hope that the teacher views this leave-taking as a positive process that frees him or her to explore another profession and be successful in it.

We have more to say about the roles of teacher evaluation in clinical supervision in chapter 5. The techniques presented there are described in terms of how they can be used to promote teacher growth; a bit of reflection will enable you to see their application to teacher evaluation. Planning and feedback conferences can be used to identify and share evaluative criteria. Classroom observation data can be used not only as feedback to the teacher but also as the basis for objective evaluation of the teacher's performance. This approach to teacher evaluation is discussed in more detail elsewhere.[10]

The Need for Clinical Supervision

Is it necessary to make clinical supervision available to teachers? This question is worth asking, especially so because research findings raise doubts about the value of this kind of supervision.

The need for clinical supervision can be defended by considering another question, "Do students need teachers?" Most educators would answer in the affirmative. All students need a teacher's assistance at one time or another; some students need more assistance than others. Very few students are so independent that they can learn solely by studying curriculum materials.

Teachers are in a similar situation. They, too, are learners. The content they need to learn is the profession of teaching. At various points in their professional development they need the skillful assistance of a clinical supervisor if they are to make progress.

In many instances the interventions of a clinical supervisor have made a significant impact on a teacher's growth. We recall a preservice teacher no one thought would survive student teaching. Continuous supervision of her classroom performance and consultation with school personnel helped her overcome feelings of insecurity and learn appropriate role behaviors.

Clinical supervision can also make a difference for an inservice teacher. We recall a teacher who was on probationary status because of low ratings on teaching effectiveness. A sympathetic supervisor helped the teacher through this difficult period, with the result that he eventually was taken off probationary status. It would have been almost impossible for that teacher to pull himself up by his own bootstraps. The supervisor's intervention was critical.

A less serious case involved an experienced primary grade teacher who had difficulty after accepting an invitation to teach a class of sixth graders. The supervisor assigned to help her quickly discovered that the teacher was trying to teach the sixth-grade class in the same manner that she had taught her second-grade classes. The supervisor collected observational data that helped the teacher see that her lesson plans and verbal behaviors were too simple for her new instructional situation. With the supervisor's assistance, the teacher was able to adjust her teaching style so that both she and the class felt more satisfied.

The Clinical Supervisor

Any educator responsible for the professional development of teachers can use the techniques of clinical supervision; methods instructors, practicum supervisors, student teaching supervisors, cooperating teachers,[11] and school administrators, to varying degrees guide the development of preservice teachers. All these educators can make use of clinical supervision techniques.

Bruce Joyce and his colleagues estimate that as many as a quarter of a million persons in the United States provide inservice education to teachers on a full-time or part-time basis.[12] These educators include 80,000 education professors, supervisors, and consultants; 100,000 principals and vice principals; and perhaps 50,000 support personnel such as reading instructors, media experts, and mental health specialists. Each of these professionals, at one time or another, may hold conferences with individual teachers or visit their classrooms for the purpose of making observations. Anyone who interacts with teachers in these contexts may find it necessary or useful to employ the techniques of clinical supervision.

Are clinical techniques useful to those whose primary or only responsibility is the evaluation of teachers? The answer is, "Yes under certain conditions." If the evaluator intends to use classroom observation data as a basis for the evaluation, the observation techniques in chapters 6–9 will be useful. If the evaluator wishes to involve the teacher in determining the criteria for evaluation, the conference techniques in chapters 3–5 will facilitate this process.

We may seem to be promoting clinical supervision as a panacea to be used by all supervisors with all teachers. To a certain extent this is true. As you become familiar with the techniques of clinical supervision you will find that they deal with basic processes—speaking, listening, influencing, observing—that occur in any supervisory contact. Because clinical supervision is built around these processes, it has a certain universality. Not all supervisors will use the "full" model of clinical supervision, however, and some will do so only under certain conditions. Other supervisors, perhaps those who see their primary role as counselor or curriculum specialist, will use only a few techniques from the clinical supervision model.

How Effective Is Clinical Supervision?

Educators ask three important questions about the effectiveness of clinical supervision:

1. Do teachers and supervisors have a positive attitude toward the clinical supervision model? Do they like it? Is it what they want?
2. Does clinical supervision result in improved teaching in the classroom?
3. Does clinical supervision result in improved learning by the teacher's students?

This section briefly considers the research relating to each question. The discussion is necessarily brief because relatively little research has been done on teacher supervision. The available research has been characterized by Richard Weller as "unsystematic, unrelated to other research, globally evaluative, and of very limited scope."[13]

Attitudes Toward Clinical Supervision

Arthur Blumberg and Edmund Amidon studied the reactions of a large group of inservice teachers to supervisory conferences with their principals.[14] Specifically, they were interested in how teachers perceived supervisors' use of "direct" behaviors (e.g., giving of information, directions or commands, and criticism) and "indirect" behaviors (e.g., accepting feelings and ideas, praise and encouragement, and asking questions). The researchers attempted to relate these perceptions of direct and indirect supervisory behavior to the same teachers' ratings of conference effectiveness.

Blumberg and Amidon found that supervisors who emphasized indirect behaviors tended to receive high ratings from teachers on the productivity of their conferences. Teachers valued indirect supervisory conferences. As indirect communication is a major element in clinical supervision, we infer that teachers would be favorable to this model of supervision (see techniques of indirect communication in chapter 5).

James Shinn's research study asked a large sample of inservice teachers to rate the ideal frequency with which they would like school principals to use various techniques of clinical supervision and the actual frequency of such use (see figure 1.2).[15] The most significant finding is that teachers believe all the techniques of clinical supervision are worthwhile: each technique was rated as meriting occasional or frequent use. The data also confirm Blumberg and Amidon's findings: several of the highest-rated techniques (e.g., 29, 30, 31) are indirect supervisory behaviors.

A study by Gary Martin provides further evidence of teachers' acceptance of the clinical supervision model.[16] Martin surveyed a group of inservice teachers and supervisors trained in the systematic observation techniques (see chapters 6–9). A comparison group of teachers and supervisors had not received this training. Martin found that the trained teachers believed their annual evaluation was more helpful to them than did the untrained teachers. Also, the trained teachers were more likely to accept evaluation as a basis for promotion and tenure decisions than were the untrained teachers. Although Martin's study focused on teacher evaluation, the findings suggest that teachers also would have a positive attitude toward the observation component of clinical supervision.

Interestingly enough, no research on supervisors' attitudes toward clinical supervision seems to have been done. There are no "hard" data on how well supervisors like clinical supervision. Nevertheless, in our experience and the experience of colleagues in conducting workshops on clinical supervision, the workshops have been well received by thousands of school principals, teacher educators, and others who have participated in them. Of course, these are informal observations that should be confirmed by systematic research.

Effects of Clinical Supervision on Teaching

Does clinical supervision help teachers improve their performance in the classroom? Norman Boyan and Willis Copeland developed an extensive training program for supervisors based on the clinical supervision model.[17] They found that supervisors trained in the model were able to help teachers make significant improvements in a variety of teaching behaviors.

In a study cited earlier, Blumberg and Amidon related teacher perceptions of supervisors' direct and indirect behaviors in conferences to teacher perceptions of learning outcomes.[18] The researchers made an interesting discovery: teachers felt they learned most about them-

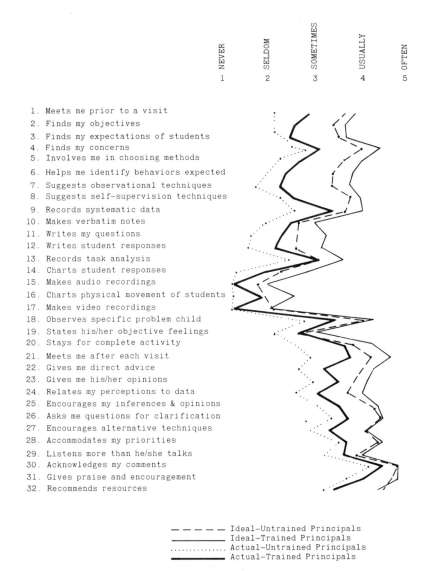

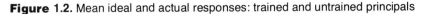

Figure 1.2. Mean ideal and actual responses: trained and untrained principals

selves, as teachers and as individuals, from conferences high in indirect *and* direct supervision.

Indirect support for clinical supervision's effectiveness can be found in the research literature on microteaching, which is a widely

used set of techniques for training teachers.[19] Microteaching techniques parallel key techniques in clinical supervision. For example, in
microteaching the teacher seeks to improve specific, operationally
defined teaching skills; in clinical supervision the supervisor helps the
teacher translate general teaching concerns into specific, observable
behaviors (technique 2). Another key ingredient of microteaching is
that the teacher presents a lesson in which he or she practices several
teaching skills. This lesson is recorded on audiotape or videotape,
then played back so that the teacher can receive feedback on the
teaching performance. The practice and feedback techniques of
microteaching are paralleled by the classroom observation (techniques 8–21) and feedback phases (techniques 22–25) of clinical
supervision. Many research studies have demonstrated that
microteaching is effective in helping teachers improve specific teaching skills. It seems reasonable to infer that if the clinical supervisor
uses techniques parallel to microteaching, similar improvements in
teaching performance will be obtained.

Effects of Clinical Supervision on Students

Ultimately, clinical supervision should improve student learning.
The clinical supervisor believes that if he (or she) can improve teacher
performance, the teacher in turn will be able to improve student
performance. If clinical supervision is effective, we should be able to
observe its effects in the supervised teacher's students. Improvements in student attitude, classroom behavior, and scholastic
achievement represent the range of possible student effects.

Unfortunately, we have not been able to locate any research on
student effects associated with clinical supervision. A possible reason
for the lack of research is the time span required to observe effects.
Such research would require a group of supervisors who would use
the clinical supervision model with a group of teachers. After supervision had occurred for a period of time, the researcher would look for
possible improvements in teacher performance. After more time had
elapsed, the researcher would look for possible improvements in student performance. The research would be costly, but it is methodo-
logically feasible.

Indirect evidence suggests that good clinical supervision results
ultimately in improved student performance. Chapter 2 presents
teaching techniques researchers have found to be associated with
student learning. For example, students of teachers who emphasize

teaching behaviors such as praise and encouragement tend to learn more than students of teachers who emphasize criticism and punishment. If clinical supervision focuses on these techniques, and if teachers show improvement in their use, then we have reason to expect that students, too, will benefit.

In summary, the links between clinical supervision and teacher performance, and between clinical supervision and student performance, have not been convincingly demonstrated. Although indirect evidence suggests that these linkages exist, research directly focused on the clinical supervision process should be encouraged.

Notes

1. Kimball Wiles, *Supervision for Better Schools*, 3rd ed. (Englewood Cliffs, NJ: Prentice-Hall, 1967).
2. Morris L. Cogan, *Supervision at the Harvard-Newton Summer School* (Cambridge, MA: Harvard Graduate School of Education, 1961).
3. Arthur Blumberg, *Supervisors and Teachers: A Private Cold War* (Berkeley, CA: McCutchan, 1974).
4. Their work is described in several books: Robert Goldhammer, *Clinical Supervision* (New York: Holt, Rinehart and Winston, 1969); Ralph L. Mosher and David E. Purpel, *Supervision: The Reluctant Profession* (Boston: Houghton Mifflin, 1972); Morris L. Cogan, *Clinical Supervision* (Boston: Houghton Mifflin, 1973).
5. Goldhammer, *Clinical Supervision*, p. 54.
6. Carl R. Rogers, *Client-Centered Therapy* (Boston: Houghton Mifflin, 1951).
7. Richard H. Weller, *Verbal Communication in Instructional Supervision* (New York: Teachers College Press, 1971).
8. Ibid., pp. 19–20. The list is reproduced here as it appears in Weller's text except that items pertaining to group clinical supervision have been omitted.
9. A poignant description of the conflicts caused by the teacher's dual role is presented in Susan Edgerton, "Teacher in Role Conflict: The Hidden Dilemma," *Phi Delta Kappan* 59 (1977): pp. 120–22.
10. Nield Oldham, *Evaluating Teachers for Professional Growth: Current Trends in School Policies and Programs* (Arlington, VA: National School Public Relations Association, 1974).
11. By "cooperating teacher" we mean a classroom teacher who supervises a preservice intern.
12. Bruce R. Joyce et al., *Inservice Teacher Education Report I: Issues to Face* (Palo Alto: Stanford Center for Research and Development in Teaching, 1967).
13. Weller, *Verbal Communication*, p. 20.
14. Arthur Blumberg and Edmund Amidon, "Teacher Perceptions of Supervisor-Teacher Interaction," *Administrators Notebook* 14 (1965): 1–8.
15. James L. Shinn, "Teacher Perceptions of Ideal and Actual Supervisory Procedures Used by California Elementary Principals: The Effects of Supervisory Training Programs Sponsored by the Association of California School Administrators" (Ph.D. diss., University of Oregon, 1976).

16. Gary S. Martin, "Teacher and Administrator Attitudes toward Evaluation and Systematic Classroom Observation" (Ph.D. diss., University of Oregon, 1975).
17. Norman J. Boyan and Willis D. Copeland, "A Training Program for Supervisors: Anatomy of an Educational Development," *Journal of Educational Research* 68 (1974): 100–116.
18. Blumberg and Amidon, "Teacher Perceptions."
19. The research literature on microteaching and related techniques has been summarized by several reviewers: W. R. Borg, M. L. Kelly, P. Langer, and M. Gall, *The Minicourse: A Microteaching Approach to Teacher Education* (Beverly Hills, CA: Macmillan Educational Services, 1970); Robert F. Peck and James A. Tucker, "Research on Teacher Education," in *Second Handbook of Research on Teaching*, ed. R. M. W. Travers (Chicago: Rand McNally, 1973), pp. 940–78.

1. pre observation conference   (planning)
2. observation
3. analysis & strategy
4. post observation conference   (feedback)
5. post conference assessment

2

Clinical Supervision and Effective Teaching

"They who educate children well are more to be honored than they who produce them."—Aristotle

We define supervision as the process of helping the teacher reduce the discrepancy between *actual* teaching behavior and *ideal* teaching behavior.[1] In this view of supervision it is important for teachers and supervisors to develop a definition of what they mean by "ideal," or effective, teaching. A good definition provides a basis for setting supervision goals and assessing their attainment.

Some educators claim that effective teaching cannot be defined because the criteria differ for every instructional situation and every teacher. They add that good teaching is so complex or so creative that it defies analysis. Some supervisors say that they cannot define good teaching but can recognize it when they see it. We are sympathetic to these views, but our experience suggests that teachers and supervisors can develop serviceable definitions of good teaching to guide the supervisory process.

As a start, we suggest that you list five characteristics of a good elementary, secondary, or college teacher.[2] Educators find this task relatively easy to perform. Moreover, they usually agree with one another's lists. Rarely do we find a controversial characteristic, that is, a characteristic some educators think is representative of good teaching and other educators think is representative of bad teaching. Disagreement, if it occurs, usually concerns the relative importance of characteristics.

Here is a list of characteristics of good teaching generated in a workshop on teacher supervision. To what extent do these characteristics agree with your list?

Characteristics of Good Teaching

- Has positive relationships with students
- Deals with students' emotions
- Maintains discipline and control
- Creates a favorable environment for learning
- Recognizes and provides for individual differences
- Enjoys working with students
- Obtains students' involvement in learning
- Is creative and innovative
- Emphasizes teaching of reading skills
- Gives students a good self-image
- Engages in professional growth activities
- Knows subject matter in depth
- Is flexible
- Is consistent
- Displays fairness

In developing your list you may wish to examine characteristics that have interested teacher educators and researchers of teacher effectiveness. A review of their work is included in this chapter, which is organized around four different perspectives for observing what teachers do. Most of the discussion is centered on the first perspective (observation of teacher behavior) because this perspective is most closely associated with the goals of clinical supervision.

Observation of Teacher Behavior

General Characteristics

The first perspective for identifying characteristics of effective teaching is to examine what teachers do in the classroom. General criteria identified by this approach are listed below under the names of the principal researchers who identified them.

Observable Indicators of Effective Classroom Teaching

Ryans's Factors
1. Teacher is warm and understanding versus cold and aloof.
2. Teacher is organized and businesslike versus unplanned and slipshod.
3. Teacher is stimulating and imaginative versus dull and routine.

Flanders's Indicators of Indirect Teaching Style
1. Teacher asks questions.
2. Teacher accepts students' feelings.
3. Teacher acknowledges students' ideas.
4. Teacher praises and encourages students.

Rosenshine and Furst's Correlates
1. Teacher is enthusiastic.
2. Teacher is businesslike and task-oriented.
3. Teacher is clear when presenting instructional content.
4. Teacher uses a variety of instructional materials and procedures.
5. Teacher provides opportunities for students to learn the instructional content.

The first three criteria of effective teaching are drawn from the work of David Ryans.[3] Ryans and his colleagues conducted an extensive program of observational studies to identify factors associated with effective teaching. Three main factors emerged from their work. The positive and negative poles of these factors are defined by (1) warm and understanding versus cold and aloof, (2) organized and businesslike versus unplanned and slipshod, and (3) stimulating and imaginative versus dull and routine. Teachers rated nearer the positive poles of each factor are considered more "effective" than teachers rated nearer the negative poles.

Another major set of research studies on teacher effectiveness is the work of Ned Flanders and his associates.[4] Flanders's studies observe two contrasting styles of teaching: direct and indirect. Direct teaching is characterized by teacher reliance on lecture, criticism, justification of authority, and giving of directions. Indirect teaching is characterized by teacher reliance on asking questions, accepting students' feelings, acknowledging students' ideas, and giving praise and encouragement.

A substantial number of studies have found that students of "indirect" teachers learn more and have better attitudes toward learning than students of "direct" teachers.[5] Flanders suggests, though, that direct *and* indirect behaviors are necessary in good teaching. For example, teachers can promote learning by a direct teaching strategy, such as lecture-explanation, to clarify a difficult curriculum topic. Even in this situation, however, the teacher can make the lecture-explanation more indirect by asking questions occasionally to determine whether students are following the presentation.

Researchers have studied teacher characteristics other than direct and indirect teaching. The usual design of these studies is to observe various aspects of teachers' classroom behavior. Also, the students of these teachers are tested at intervals during the school year. Standardized achievement tests frequently are used for this purpose. The students' scores before and after a period of instruction (e.g., at the beginning and end of a school year) are compared to obtain a measure of "achievement gain." Finally, the data are analyzed to determine which teacher behaviors are associated with student achievement gains.

Barak Rosenshine and Norma Furst have done a useful review of these research studies.[6] They identified five teacher characteristics consistently associated with gains in student achievement. (By "associated" we mean that teachers with "more" of the particular characteristic tend to have higher-achieving students than teachers with "less" of the characteristic.) The first two characteristics are teacher enthusiasm and businesslike orientation, characteristics also identified in Ryans's research. The third characteristic is teacher clarity. Researchers have defined clarity, or the lack of it, in various ways— for example, the amount of time the teacher uses to answer student questions requesting clarification of what the teacher said; the frequency with which students respond to a teacher's questions without the teacher needing to intersperse additional information or questions; and the avoidance of vague words (e.g., "some," "many," "of course") in the teacher's oral discourse.

The fourth Rosenshine and Furst teacher characteristic is variety in teaching. This characteristic can be observed by counting the number of different instructional materials, tests, and teaching devices used by the teacher. Another indicator is the extent to which the teacher varies the cognitive level of classroom discourse.

The fifth characteristic is the extent to which the teacher provides opportunities for students to learn the curriculum material covered by the achievement tests. In a sense, this characteristic reflects the extent to which the teacher "teaches to the test." However, we can view this characteristic as the teacher's ability and preference for classroom activities focused on the kinds of cognitive learning usually measured by achievement tests.

Subject Matter: Specific Criteria

In recent years researchers have made a concerted effort to identify teacher behaviors that facilitate student learning in specific curriculum areas. Much of this research has focused on reading and mathematics instruction at the primary and elementary school levels.

Barak Rosenshine summarized and interpreted the major recent research on teacher behaviors related to success in reading and mathematics instruction in primary-level, low-socioeconomic-status classrooms.[7] These behaviors, which are listed below, form a pattern Rosenshine labels "direct instruction."

Rosenshine's List of Teacher Behaviors Related to Effective Reading and Mathematics Instruction[8]

1. Classroom time is structured by the teacher.
2. Teacher devotes classroom time to reading and mathematics instruction by means of textbooks, academic workbooks, and verbal interaction.
3. Teacher assigns seatwork involving academic workbooks through which students work at their own pace.
4. Teacher organizes students into small groups and supervises their work.
5. Teacher directs activities without giving students choice of activities or reasons for the selection of activities.
6. Teacher asks direct questions that have only a single answer.
7. Teacher encourages students to attempt to answer questions, even when they say they don't know the answers.
8. Teacher immediately reinforces students on the accuracy of their answers.
9. Teacher asks a new question after student has given a correct answer.
10. Teacher gives the correct answer after a student has given an incorrect answer.

Direct instruction differs from the inquiry-oriented methods and open classroom approach sometimes recommended for primary school instruction. In contrast to these other methods, direct instruction calls for the teacher to structure students' time rather than let students structure their own time; to emphasize small-group work rather than independent learning; to engage in frequent drill rather than encourage student self-expression; and to give frequent, immediate feedback to students' answers. The research reviewed by Rosenshine suggests that the reading and mathematics achievement of primary-grade, low-SES students can be improved if the teacher uses this highly directive teaching pattern.

David Berliner and William Tikunoff conducted a large-scale research study in which they attempted to identify teacher behaviors that discriminated between more effective and less effective teachers in second-grade reading, second-grade mathematics, fifth-grade reading, and fifth-grade mathematics.[9] Teacher effectiveness was defined in terms of student gain on standardized achievement tests that measured the content of curriculum units constructed for each grade level and subject area.

Berliner and Tikunoff identified twenty-one teacher behaviors that discriminated between more effective and less effective teachers at each grade level and subject area. These behaviors are listed below. As you can see, the list is in two parts: teacher behaviors that contribute to student learning, and teacher behaviors that detract from it. This list is surprisingly consistent with the findings of Ryans, Flanders, and Rosenshine and Furst.

Berliner and Tikunoff's List of Teacher Behaviors Related to Effective Reading and Mathematics Instruction

Effective Teacher Behaviors
1. Teacher reacts constructively (overt, verbal, nonverbal) to students' feelings and attitudes.
2. Teacher actively listens to what a student is saying, reading, reciting.
3. Teacher gives a direction or a threat and follows through with it.
4. Teacher seems confident in teaching a given subject and demonstrates a grasp of it.
5. Teacher checks in on student's progress regularly and adjusts instruction accordingly.

6. Teacher expresses positive, pleasant, optimistic attitudes and feelings.
7. Teacher seems to perceive learning rate of students and adjusts teaching pace accordingly.
8. Teacher encourages students to take responsibility for their own classwork.
9. Teacher capitalizes instructionally on unexpected incidents that arise during class time.
10. Teacher prepares students for lesson by reviewing, outlining, explaining objectives, and summarizing.

Ineffective Teacher Behaviors
1. Teacher switches abruptly, e.g., from instruction to classroom management.
2. Teacher berates child in front of others.
3. Teacher fills "empty" time periods with "busywork."
4. Teacher makes a statement whose consequences would be ridiculous if carried out.
5. Teacher often treats whole group as "one" in order to maintain peer control.
6. Teacher calls attention to self for no apparent instructional purpose.

Teaching Strategies

In the preceding section we discussed a variety of general teacher characteristics that can be assessed by observing teachers' classroom performance. It also is possible to observe teachers' use of more specific strategies and techniques. Discussion, lecture, inquiry, recitation, diagnostic-prescriptive teaching, behavior modification, independent learning contracts, simulations, and role playing are examples of teaching strategies that competent teachers might be expected to have in their repertoire. Research has demonstrated the effectiveness of each of these teaching strategies in promoting certain types of learning, although the evidence is not always conclusive.[10]

Each teaching strategy can be analyzed further into a set of techniques. For example, some techniques viewed as desirable in recitations are (1) asking higher cognitive questions rather than knowledge-level questions exclusively, (2) pausing after asking a question to allow students time to think, (3) asking follow-up questions to help students improve their original response to a question, and (4) distributing participation among students evenly.

Teachers can be observed and rated on their overall effectiveness in using this strategy and also on their effectiveness in using each technique.

Every major teaching strategy has several variants and specialized applications in different curriculum fields. For example, the discussion method can take different forms, depending on whether the teacher uses it to promote higher cognitive learning, clarification of issues, or problem solving. Subject-matter specialists also have adapted this method for their use. In social studies Oliver and Shaver have developed a variant of the discussion method that supports their jurisprudential model for analyzing public issues.[11] Chapter 4 presents procedures for observing strategies and techniques frequently recommended by educators.

Observation of the Teacher's Students

The second perspective for examining quality of teaching is to observe the teacher's students. Even without knowing anything about a teacher, a supervisor can make judgments about the quality of his or her teaching by observing the teacher's students. Observable aspects of student behavior and performance are listed below.

Observable Indicators of Effective Teaching: Student Behavior and Performance

1. Students are learning the knowledge, understandings, skills, and attitudes intended by the curriculum, as measured by performance on tests.
2. Students exhibit independent behavior in learning the curriculum.
3. Students exhibit behaviors that indicate a positive attitude toward the teacher and their peers.
4. Students exhibit behaviors that indicate a positive attitude toward the curriculum and the school.
5. Students exhibit behaviors that indicate a positive attitude toward themselves as learners.
6. Students do not exhibit behavior problems in class.

7.   Students seem actively engaged in learning the curriculum while class is in session.

Supervisors can examine test results to determine how well students are learning the curriculum, either over a short unit of study or over a school year. They can observe whether students exhibit behaviors that indicate a positive attitude toward varied aspects of schooling and whether students are well behaved during class activities.

Indicator 7 in the list is of particular importance. Barak Rosenshine and David Berliner, in a review of recent research on teaching, have concluded that *academic engaged time* is an important factor in school achievement.[12] By academic engaged time, Rosenshine and Berliner mean the amount of time a student spends in reading, writing, manipulating. or other activities that engage the student in learning academically relevant material. In their review they found that amount of academic engaged time in reading and math activities was positively associated with student achievement in these subjects. In other words, the more time, the more achievement. Time spent on other activities was *negatively* associated with student achievement.

Academic engaged time seems an important factor in student learning. The "at task" method (technique 11) provides a good observational measure of this factor.

Observation of the Teacher's Planning

The third perspective for developing criteria of good teaching is the teacher's planning. It is easy to misjudge the effectiveness of a teacher's classroom behavior unless you know the teacher's intent and instructional objectives. For example, we recall a group of educators who observed a sixth-grade teacher conducting a question-and-answer session with her class. Afterward, one of the group criticized the teacher for asking too many knowledge-level questions. The teacher later met with the group and explained that the class needed the question-and-answer session to reinforce the information contained in a difficult lesson the preceding day. The teacher further explained that she intended to have another lesson in which students would be encouraged to reflect on, and apply, their newly acquired information. In brief, one of the educators had misjudged the teacher's classroom performance because he did not know the teacher's intent.

There are several possible indicators of quality in the teacher's planning efforts. It is possible to judge the soundness of the teachers' rationale in choosing instructional objectives, curriculum materials, and evaluation techniques. The teacher's rationale can be determined by talking with the teacher and examining the written lesson plans.

Another important aspect of the teacher's planning is use of student characteristics and ability to organize and individualize instruction. Evidence of good planning is also found in the teacher's approach to revising instructional plans, if necessary, based on the outcome of classroom performance.

In chapter 3 we emphasize again the need in supervision to determine the teacher's plans and intents (techniques 1–7). Without knowing them, the supervisor is likely to misjudge the effectiveness of the teacher's classroom behavior. In contrast, knowledge of a teacher's plans and intent enables the supervisor to help the teacher analyze how well his or her actual classroom behavior corresponded to what was planned.

Observation of the Teacher Outside the Classroom

The teacher's performance in settings other than the classroom provides the fourth major basis for developing criteria of good teaching. These criteria include the effectiveness with which the teacher participates in school activities, cooperates with colleagues, and engages in professional growth activities. The extent to which the teacher's behavior conforms to ethical norms sometimes is considered a criterion of good teaching. Additional criteria can be listed—for example, the effectiveness of the teacher's participation in curriculum selection committees. At colleges and universities, research publication and service to the profession frequently are criteria for judging the teacher's effectiveness.

Developing a Definition of Effective Teaching

The preceding discussion was not intended to provide a comprehensive definition of "good" teaching. You may disagree with some or all of the criteria presented. Our main purpose was to present perspectives from which you can develop your own definition of effective teaching. Another purpose was to acquaint you with the findings of recent research on teacher effectiveness.

We suggest that you, in your role as teacher supervisor, find time to create a personal definition of effective teaching. It is also important for teachers under supervision to develop a definition. Some supervisors and teachers have different, even conflicting, definitions of good teaching. Their definitions may include the same characteristics but differ in the relative importance they attribute to them. For example, some teachers and supervisors place greatest value on the teacher's ability to improve students' self-concepts. Other teachers and supervisors value most the teacher's ability to promote students' learning of the 3 Rs. Chapter 5 discusses how these differences in perspective can interfere with effective supervision unless they are acknowledged and resolved.

Notes

1. Some educators prefer the terms "good" or "effective" rather than "ideal." We use these terms interchangeably in the text.
2. You can elaborate on this task by listing five or more characteristics of an ineffective teacher.
3. D. G. Ryans, *Characteristics of Teachers* (Washington, DC: American Council on Teachers, 1960).
4. Ned A. Flanders, *Analyzing Teaching Behavior* (Reading, MA: Addison-Wesley, 1970).
5. J. R. Campbell and C. W. Barnes, "Interaction Analysis—A Breakthrough?" *Phi Delta Kappan* 50 (1969): 587–90. But see also Barrak Rosenshine, "Interaction Analysis: A Tardy Comment," *Phi Delta Kappan* 51 (1970): 445–46.
6. Barak Rosenshine and Norma F. Furst, "Research on Teacher Performance Criteria," in *Research in Teacher Education: A Symposium*, ed. B. O. Smith (Englewood Cliffs, NJ: Prentice-Hall, 1971), 37–72.
7. Barak Rosenshine, "Classroom Instruction," in *The Psychology of Teaching Methods: The Seventy-Fifth Yearbook of the National Society for the Study of Education*, ed. N. L. Gage (Chicago: University of Chicago Press, 1976), 335–71.
8. List is adapted from ibid., 369–70.
9. David C. Berliner and William J. Tikunoff, "The California Beginning Teacher Evaluation Study: Overview of the Ethnographic Study," *Journal of Teacher Education*, 27 (1976): 24–30.
10. Much of this research is summarized in N. L. Gage, ed., *The Psychology of Teaching Methods*; and N. L. Gage and David C. Berliner, *Educational Psychology* (Chicago: Rand McNally, 1975).
11. This discussion model is described in Marsha Weil and Bruce Joyce, *Social Models of Teaching: Expanding Your Teaching Repertoire* (Englewood Cliffs, NJ: Prentice-Hall, 1978), pp. 109–80.
12. Barak V. Rosenshine and David C. Berliner, "Academic Engaged Time," *British Journal of Teacher Education* 4 (1978): 3–16.

Unit Exercises

Multiple-Choice Items

Answers are on page 192.

1. Clinical supervision includes these sequential stages:

    a. planning conference, feedback conference, classroom observation.

    b. classroom observation, feedback conference, planning conference.

    c. planning conference, classroom observation, feedback conference.

    d. counseling conference, classroom observation, feedback conference.

2. Research has shown that teachers:

    a. are satisfied with supervision as currently practiced.

    b. believe that supervision plays an important role in their professional lives.

    c. look to supervision primarily for emotional support and reassurance.

    d. hold supervision in low regard.

3. The major purpose of clinical supervision is:

    a. to improve the teacher's classroom instruction.

    b. to provide curriculum support to the teacher.

    c. to provide emotional support and reassurance to the teacher.

    d. (*b*) and (*c*) are correct.

4. The techniques of clinical supervision:

    a. should never be used in teacher evaluation.

    b. can be adapted for use in teacher evaluation.

    c. can be used in teacher evaluation, except for the techniques of the feedback conference.

    d. can be used in teacher evaluation, except for the techniques of the planning conference.

5. Which of the following generalizations is best supported by the available research evidence?

37

    ₀ a.   Teachers prefer an indirect supervisory style.
      b.   Teachers prefer a direct supervisory style.
      c.   Clinical supervision results in improved learning by the
           teacher's students.
      d.   Clinical supervision results in improved teacher retention by
           school districts.

6.   Which of the following indicators has *not* been found to be a
     correlate of effective teaching?

      a.   Teacher warmth
      b.   Teacher enthusiasm
    ₐ c.   Teacher experience
      d.   Teacher clarity

7.   Of the perspectives for observing what teachers do, which is the
     most closely associated with the goals of clinical supervision?

      a.   Observation of the teacher outside the classroom
      b.   Observation of the teacher's students
      c.   Observation of the teacher's planning
    ᵥ d.   Observation of the teacher's classroom behavior

8.   The behaviors of accepting students' feelings, acknowledging
     student ideas, and praising students are indicators of

      a.   teacher task-orientation.
      b.   teacher clarity.
      c.   academic engaged time.
    ₐ d.   indirect teaching style.

Problems

   The following problems do not have single correct answers. Possible answers are on pages 192–93. Your answers may differ from ours
yet be as good or better.

1.   As a clinical supervisor, you are working with a teacher to help
     her develop new skills as she makes the transition from high
     school teaching to junior high school teaching. One day the
     teacher becomes distressed and says she is considering leaving
     the profession. What do you do in your role as clinical super-
     visor?
2.   You are assigned to be the clinical supervisor of an undergraduate

who is just starting a student-teaching placement. The under-graduate initiates a conversation with you by asking, "Are you here to evaluate me?" How might you respond?

3. Some educators claim that good teachers are born, not made. Others claim that teaching can never be analyzed because it is an art, not a science. Do you agree or disagree with these claims? Why?

Unit II

Techniques of Clinical Conferences

Overview

Two of the three stages of the clinical supervision process require conferences between the supervisor and the teacher: planning and feedback. Chapter 3 considers the essentials of an effective planning conference, chapter 4 deals with techniques for providing useful feedback to teachers, and chapter 5 compares direct and indirect approaches to conference strategies or styles of supervision. Specific techniques are described with examples of how they can be used to make conferences productive.

Objectives

The purpose of this unit is to help you develop:

Understanding of the basic elements of a positive relationship between the supervisor and the teacher.

Specific steps for conducting a conference in which teacher and supervisor plan cooperatively to address specific concerns, observe and record behavior, and work together to improve instruction.

Explicit techniques for providing useful feedback to teachers to aid them in analyzing, interpreting, and modifying their instructional efforts.

An approach to supervision consistent in style, strategy, and technique with the goals set forth in unit 1.

3

The Planning
Conference

"The most important link between a teacher and his supervisor
is effective communication. . . . The principal must set the stage
for open communication. Teachers see the justification for
supervision and evaluation programs, but they want to be a
partner in the process."—Robert L. Herchberger and James M.
Young, Jr., "Teacher Perceptions of Supervision and Evaluation"

The planning conference sets the stage for effective clinical supervision. It provides the teacher and supervisor with an opportunity to identify teacher concerns and translate them into observable behaviors. Another outcome of the planning conference is a decision about the kinds of instructional data that will be recorded during
classroom observation, which is the next phase of the supervisory
cycle.

The planning conference is organized around an agenda that calls
for the identification of teacher concerns, possible solutions to these
concerns, and observation techniques. Less obvious but no less important are certain processes that occur in the conference. For example, during the planning conference the teacher may decide how
much trust to place in the supervisor. Trust refers to the teacher's
confidence that the supervisor has the teacher's interests at heart and
that the supervisor will not use data that emerge during supervision

against the teacher. Supervisors may be technically proficient, but unless they also instill trust, their supervision is likely to be inefficient. We have more to say about trust-instilling behaviors in chapter 5.

A basic purpose of the planning conference is to provide an opportunity for the teacher to communicate with a fellow educator about a unique classroom situation and style of teaching. Many teachers feel isolated in their work because they usually teach alone in a self-contained classroom. By periodically observing the teacher's classroom, the supervisor builds a set of shared experiences that supervisor and teacher can discuss together in their conferences. These conferences are especially important to the student teacher who may have no one in the school other than the supervisor with whom to share concerns and perceptions.

Planning conferences need not be long. As a supervisor, you might allow twenty to thirty minutes for the first planning conference unless the teacher has a particularly difficult problem to discuss. Later planning conferences might require only five to ten minutes, especially if there has been no change in the teacher's goals for improvement since the preceeding clinical supervision cycle of planning-observation-feedback.

Planning conferences probably are best held on neutral territory (e.g., the school cafeteria, if it is free) or in the teacher's classroom. Going into a supervisor's office for a conference may be perceived by the teacher as being "called on the carpet."

This chapter presents seven techniques to use in the planning conference. These techniques constitute an agenda for the conference. In fact, you should consider using them in the order in which they are presented.

These techniques are important for a successful planning conference, yet we also acknowledge their limitations. A supervisor may use all these techniques and still not have a satisfactory conference because some other element (e.g., teacher's trust) is missing. There may be conference techniques that we have overlooked. Also, the techniques presented here are not highly specific prescriptions. You will need to use judgment in incorporating them into your supervisory behavior and in applying them to a particular supervisory situation. Our only claim is that judicious use of these techniques provides a sound base for conducting a planning conference. What you as a person contribute to this base is critical for success.

This chapter concludes with the transcript of an actual planning conference that incorporates the seven conference techniques.

Identify the Teacher's Concerns About Instruction (Technique 1)

The major purpose of clinical supervision is to help teachers improve their classroom instruction. One step toward this goal is to use the planning conference to identify areas of instruction in which a teacher needs improvement.

A supervisor might directly ask a teacher in what ways he or she would like to improve as a teacher, but this is not usually effective. Many teachers have not formulated self-improvement goals and feel put on the spot when asked to do so. A more useful approach initially is to assist the teacher in identifying concerns. A teacher who can identify and verbalize concerns can usually take the next steps of examining the concerns objectively and solving them.

There are a variety of questions that a supervisor might ask to guide the teacher's thinking about concerns. For example: "How has your teaching been going?" "Do you find you are having more success in one area than another?" "Our goal is to help you do the best possible teaching. Are there any aspects of your teaching we should take a look at?"

No one question is better than another. The supervisor should be intent on helping the teacher reveal true concerns without feeling threatened. A threatened teacher is likely to clam up or reveal only "safe" concerns. For example, teachers have told us that "individualization of instruction" is a safe concern, but discipline is not a safe concern. A teacher who mentions discipline problems may be perceived as incompetent, whereas a teacher who mentions individualization is likely to be perceived as well along the road toward being a master teacher.

Some teachers insist that they have no concerns; their class is running beautifully. In some instances this may be an accurate perception by the teacher, but we would suggest that there is always room for improvement in one's teaching. A good teacher can get better.

When a teacher insists that he or she has no concerns, the supervisor probably should take the statement at face value. The supervisor might also suggest using a "wide-lens" observation technique such as video recording (see chapter 8) so that they can look together at the teacher's instruction. An appropriate tone can be set by asking, "How about making a videotape of one of your lessons so that we can see what aspects of your teaching please you?" After the video recording has been made and reviewed in the feedback conference, the teacher may become aware of areas for improvement that were not previously apparent.

Sometimes teachers find it helpful to examine the checklist or other instruments that will be used to evaluate their teaching performance. In showing the checklist to a teacher, the supervisor might ask, "Which of these areas do you think you're strong in? Which of these areas do you think we might take a closer look at as areas for improvement?"

Frances Fuller did a classic series of investigations at the University of Texas on teachers' concerns during training and into their professional careers.[1] She found that the concerns of preservice teachers and new inservice teachers tend to focus on the self. The concerns of experienced teachers tend to focus on their students. Fuller summarized her findings in the following form:

EARLY TEACHING PHASE: CONCERN WITH SELF

Covert Concerns: Where do I stand? When teaching starts, [student] teachers ask themselves, "Where do I stand?" . . . "Is it going to be my class or the teacher's class?" "If I see a child misbehaving in the hall, do I handle it, ignore it, or tell someone else?" . . . These concerns were rarely expressed in either written statements or in routine interviews unless directly elicited.

Overt Concerns: How Adequate Am I? The concern student teachers feel about class control is no secret. It is a blatant persistent concern of most beginning teachers.

Ability to control the class, however, is apparently just part of a larger concern of the new teacher with his adequacy in the classroom. This larger concern involves abilities to understand subject matter, to know the answers, to say "I don't know," to have the freedom to fail on occasion, to anticipate problems, to mobilize resources and to make changes when failures reoccur. It also involves the ability to cope with evaluation: the willingness to listen for evaluation and to parcel out the biases of evaluators.

LATE CONCERNS: CONCERN WITH PUPILS

. . . When concerns are "mature," i.e., characteristic of experienced superior teachers, concerns seem to focus on pupil gain and self-evaluation as opposed to personal gain and evaluation by others. The specific concerns we have observed are concerns about ability to understand pupils' capacities, to specify objectives for them, to assess their gain, to apportion out one's own contributions to pupils' difficulties and gain, and to evaulate oneself in terms of pupil gain.[2]

Frances Fuller's insights suggest the variety of teacher concerns to which the supervisor must remain sensitive. As she notes, some of these concerns are easily verbalized by the teacher. Others must be solicited through careful questioning.

Translate the Teacher's Concerns into Observable Behaviors (Technique 2)

Helping a teacher translate concerns into observable behaviors is one of the most important techniques of clinical supervision. For an analogy, consider the patient who visits a doctor with vague complaints of not feeling well. The doctor's first task is to develop a differentiated picture of the patient's symptoms. The doctor does this by asking such questions as "How long have you felt this way?" "What are the specific problems you've been having?" "What does the discomfort feel like?" These questions are part of a diagnostic process the doctor uses, first, to isolate the problem, and then to prescribe a treatment.

The clinical supervisor similarly needs to function as a diagnostician in the planning conference. Suppose a student teacher says, "I'm not sure I have the confidence to be a teacher." The teacher's expressed concern is lack of confidence, but the supervisor needs to probe further. *Confidence* may mean something different to the teacher than it means to the supervisor.

In using the technique of translating concerns, the supervisor needs to listen for the teacher's use of words and phrases that are abstract, ambiguous, or stated at a high level of generality. These typically are concepts that are one level removed from observable behavior. The following are examples of teacher statements that contain abstract or ambiguous words:

"I'm afraid I'm a *dictator*."
"To me the most important thing is for students to have a *healthy self-concept*."
"There's just not enough time to *cover everything I want to get across*."
"Some of my students are just like *wild animals*."

"I'm afraid I don't project *warmth*."
"I wonder if I'm too *critical* of students."
"How do you *reach* these *problem* students?"

When you hear a teacher use such terms to refer to a concern, your task is to clarify the terms so that they are stated in observable form. Here are examples of questions that might help the teacher state a concern more concretely:

"Do you know a teacher who projects *warmth*? What does she do?"
"What kinds of things do you do that make you think you're *critical* of students?"
"In what ways are these *problem* students?"
"Can you clarify what you mean by *reaching* problem students?"

These are not the only kinds of questions that are useful. The supervisor is free to use any questions or other technique that help the teacher focus on abstract terms and clarify their meaning.

A supervisor can judge success in translating concerns by considering this question: "Do I have enough information so that I can clearly observe the teacher's concern as it is expressed in his classroom?" Another good question is "Do the teacher and I mean the same thing when we use the term _____?" If your answer to both questions is a confident yes, this is a good indication that you are using the technique properly.

Several research studies have been done to clarify the meaning of key concepts in teaching. For example, Andrew Bush, John Kennedy, and Donald Cruikshank conducted research to determine the observable referents of teacher *clarity*.[3] Their approach was to ask students to list five behaviors performed by their clearest teacher. They were able to identify the following observable behaviors underlying the concept of clarity:

- gives examples and explains them
- repeats questions and explanations if students don't understand them
- lets students ask questions
- pronounces words distinctly
- talks only about things related to the topic he is teaching
- uses common words
- writes important things on the blackboard
- relates what he is teaching to real life

- asks questions to find out if students understand what he has told them

Although this list is not exhaustive, it is a great help to teacher and supervisor in their efforts to improve the clarity of the teacher's instruction.

Even a nonverbal concept such as teacher enthusiasm can be made observable through careful analysis. Mary Collins identified observable referents for enthusiasm by reviewing previous research on this variable, by her own analysis, and by consulting other teacher educators.[4] Collins's list of observable behaviors is presented below. Using this list as a guide, she was able to train a group of preservice elementary teachers to improve their level of enthusiasm significantly in classroom instruction.

You will find more examples of observable referents for teacher concerns in chapters 6–9. These chapters present a collection of observation instruments for recording data about many different teacher concerns.

Observable Referents for Enthusiasm

1. Vocal Delivery: Great and sudden changes from rapid excited speech to a whisper; varied, lilting, uplifting intonations; many changes in tone, pitch
2. Eyes: Dancing, snapping, shining, lighting up, frequently opened wide, eyebrows raised, eye contact with total group
3. Gestures: Frequent demonstrative movements of body, head, arms, hands, and face; sweeping motions; clapping hands; head nodding rapidly
4. Movements: Large body movements; swings around, changes pace, bends body
5. Facial Expression: Appears vibrant, demonstrative; changes denoting surprise, sadness, joy, thoughtfulness, awe, excitement
6. Word Selection: Highly descriptive, many adjectives, great variety
7. Acceptance of Ideas and Feelings: Accepts ideas and feelings quickly with vigor and animation; ready to accept, praise, en-

courage, or clarify in a nonthreatening manner; many variations in responding to pupils

8. Overall Energy: Explosive, exuberant; high degree of vitality, drive, and spirit throughout lesson

Identify Procedures for Improving the Teacher's Instruction (Technique 3)

The first two techniques are intended to help the teacher identify concerns and translate them into observable behaviors. What happens next?

If the teacher has successfully identified some concerns, the stage is set for thinking about possible changes in instructional behavior. For example, consider a teacher who is worried that he comes across as dull and unenthusiastic. As the supervisor helps this teacher identify observable behaviors that comprise enthusiasm, the teacher is likely to ask himself, "I wonder how I could get myself to do those things." The supervisor facilitates this process by thinking aloud with the teacher about procedures he can use to acquire new behaviors.

The simplest procedure, perhaps, is for the teacher to practice the behaviors on his own. The supervisor might say, "Why don't you make a list of these enthusiasm behaviors on a five-by-eight-inch card and keep it near you when you teach? In a week or so, I'll come in and make a video recording so you can see how you're doing."

Sometimes the needed procedures are more involved. For example, one teacher's concern may be how to use learning centers effectively. This involves a whole set of instructional skills. To acquire these skills, the teacher may need to do some reading and to attend workshops on learning centers.

If a teacher's concern is about changing student behavior, a sequence of procedures is needed. To illustrate, suppose the teacher is concerned that students do not pay attention during class discussions. The supervisor first helps the teacher to define "attention" as a set of observable behaviors—answering teacher's questions thoughtfully, looking at other students as they speak, initiating relevant comments and questions, and so forth. The teacher's next task is to develop instructional procedures that will bring about these desired "attending" behaviors. Finally, the teacher will need to practice these instructional procedures until they are mastered.

In brief, three steps are involved in bringing about change in students' behavior:

1. Identify the *specific student behaviors* you (the teacher) wish your class to use.
2. Identify the *instructional procedures* you will need to use to bring about the specific student behaviors.
3. Identify a strategy for learning and practicing the instructional procedures.

Bringing about change in student behavior is probably the most difficult goal a teacher can strive for, but it also yields the greatest rewards.

The following is an excerpt from a planning conference in which the goal was change in the behavior of second-grade children:

Teacher: I'd like you to come in and take a look at Randall and Ronald. They don't do anything but play and talk.

Supervisor: Are Randall and Ronald the only ones you want me to observe?

Teacher: No. I have a real immature group this year. You might as well observe all of them.

Supervisor: What do you mean by "immature"?

Teacher: Oh, they have very short attention spans, haven't learned to settle down, and they just talk without permission.

At this point, teacher and supervisor decided to focus on one problem behavior—talking without permission. The dialogue continues.

Supervisor: Can you give an example of a situation where they talk without permission?

Teacher: Well, when I have them in a small reading group, and I ask one of them a question, any of them will speak up if they think they have the answer. Sometimes they don't even listen to the question, they just say what's on their mind. And it doesn't matter whether another child is already talking. They'll just ignore him and speak at the same time.

Supervisor: I think I have a pretty clear idea of what's happening. What do you think you can do so that only the

> child you call on responds, and so that if another
> child has something to say, he waits his turn?

Teacher: I guess I could teach them some rules for par-
ticipating. Like raising their hands when they wish
to speak and remaining quiet when another child
is speaking.

Teacher and supervisor proceeded to discuss possible methods of
teaching these rules to the children. The teacher took notes on the
procedures and agreed to practice them the following week. In addition, the supervisor suggested that the teacher try praising or otherwise rewarding children when they obey participation rules in the
reading group. In making this suggestion, the supervisor discovered
that the teacher was unfamiliar with the reinforcement principles underlying the use of praise and other rewards in classroom teaching.
The supervisor therefore suggested that the teacher might benefit
from enrolling in an upcoming workshop on classroom management
in which these principles would be discussed.

This example illustrates the three steps in bringing about change in
student behavior: (1) identify the specific student behaviors
desired—students raising hands when they wish to speak and being
silent when another child is speaking; (2) identify instructional
procedures—teaching children the instructional rules and rewarding
them for appropriate behavior; and (3) identify a strategy for learning
the instructional procedures—practice in the classroom and attending
a workshop.

Assist the Teacher in Setting Self-Improvement Goals (Technique 4)

If the supervisor has used the first three techniques effectively, it
should be relatively easy to help the teacher take the next step: setting
personal goals for improvement of instruction.

Some supervisors and teachers may feel this step is superfluous. In
discussing the previous technique, we presented the example of a
teacher concerned about students speaking out of turn The supervisor helped the teacher identify several observable behaviors of students that reflected this concern and also helped the teacher identify
procedures for changing these behaviors. It seems apparent that the
teacher's goal is to improve students' verbal participation behaviors in

reading groups. The clinical supervision process is facilitated by making this goal explicit. By doing so, teacher and supervisor both develop a clear understanding of the direction toward which the clinical supervision process is headed. It also prevents a state of confusion, with the teacher thinking, "I wonder what the supervisor expects me to be doing?"

The supervisor or the teacher can state the goal, but whoever does so should check that the other person has the same understanding of the goal and agrees with it. In the example we have been considering, the goal formulation process might occur as follows:

Supervisor:	To review, then, one of the things you're concerned about is students speaking out of turn. You've picked out a number of behaviors you'd like to see your students engage in. Given that, is there a goal you would set for yourself?
Teacher:	Yes. My first goal is to reduce the incidence of students' speaking out of turn. My other goal is to have my students engage in more positive behaviors, like listening to one another and raising their hands when they have something to say.
Supervisor:	Those are worthwhile goals, and I'll do what I can to help you with them.

This interchange between teacher and supervisor, if done naturally and genuinely, gives structure and focus to the planning conference.

Arrange a Time for Classroom Observation (Technique 5)

The first four techniques of the planning conference have involved the teacher and supervisor in *talking* about the teacher's instruction. Now it is time to plan for *observing* the instruction firsthand.

The first step in planning for observation is to arrange a mutually convenient time for the supervisor to visit the classroom. For one reason or another, there may be certain lessons the teacher does not wish you to observe or you are unable to observe because of time conflicts. The major criterion for selecting a lesson is that it should present opportunities for the teacher's concerns and solutions to those concerns. If the teacher's concern is students' responses to discussion questions, there is no point in observing a lesson in which students are engaged in independent learning projects.

Arranging a mutually convenient time for classroom observation is important for another reason. Teachers are resentful when supervisors come to their room unannounced. Teachers need to feel that the supervisor respects them as professionals and as people with first-line responsibility for their classrooms. They are not likely to feel this way if a supervisor "pops in" anytime he or she wishes to do so.

The technique of arranging a mutually convenient time is important when supervising experienced teachers, but it is equally important when working with student teachers. They can be put into a state of constant tension if they are led to think the supervisor can enter their class anytime unannounced. Arranging a time beforehand enables the student teacher to prepare instructionally (and emotionally) for the supervisor's visit. It also gives the student teacher a feeling of some control over the supervisory process. A student teacher who has this feeling of control is likely to use supervision for self-improvement rather than feel used by it.

Select an Observation Instrument and Behaviors to Be Recorded (Technique 6)

The planning conference is based on the teacher's *perceptions* of what occurs in the classroom. These perceptions may coincide or differ substantially from what actually occurs. Observational data are needed to provide an objective check on the teacher's perceptions and also to record instructional phenomena that may have escaped the teacher's attention. Therefore, an important step in the planning conference is for supervisor and teacher together to decide what kinds of observational data might be worth collecting.

A wide range of observation instruments is presented in unit 3. You will need to become familiar with them in order to help the teacher select an observation instrument appropriate for his or her instructional concerns.

The observation instrument should be matched carefully with the teacher's particular instructional concerns. For example, if a teacher is concerned about her nonverbal behavior, a video recording (technique 15) might be appropriate. If the concern is about a problem child in the classroom, an anecdotal record (technique 14) would be helpful. Or if a teacher is concerned about the level of commotion in his classroom, a record of students' movement patterns (technique 13) could be made.

The selection of an observation instrument helps sharpen a teacher's thinking about instruction. If teacher and supervisor use the conference only to *talk* about instruction, the conversation may drift off into vague generalities and abstractions. Selecting an observation instrument brings the teacher "down to earth" by focusing attention on the observable realities of classroom instruction.

Either the supervisor or the teacher can suggest appropriate observation instruments and behaviors to be recorded on them. If the teacher is unfamiliar with methods of classroom observation, the supervisor may need to initiate suggestions. Once teachers become familiar with the range of instruments, however, they should be encouraged to initiate their own suggestions.

In discussing observation instruments with teachers, you may wish to stress their nonevaluative nature. These instruments are designed to collect nonevaluative, objective data that teachers can inspect in the feedback conference and from which they can form their own judgments about the effectiveness of their teaching.

Clarify the Instructional Context in Which Data Will Be Recorded (Technique 7)

Throughout this book we emphasize the importance of focusing on one or two areas of concern at a time. A teacher who is asked to look at too many aspects of instruction at once is likely to become confused. Your classroom observation might focus on the teacher's enthusiasm, or discipline technique, or the task behavior of students. However, there is a risk that the recording of observational data will be oversimplified. Instructional behaviors do not occur in a vacuum. They occur in a context that must be understood if the target behaviors are to be interpreted properly.

In short, the supervisor cannot walk into a teacher's classroom "cold" and expect to understand what is happening. Therefore, an effective technique is to ask the teacher a few questions about the instructional context of the behaviors to be recorded. Since the usual instructional context is a lesson which the teacher plans to teach, you may wish to ask the teacher such questions as:

"What is the lesson about that I'll be observing?"
"What do you expect the students to learn in this lesson?"
"What strategy will you be using?"
"Is there anything I should be aware of as you teach this lesson?"

Asking these questions indicates to the teacher that you wish to understand the teacher's "world" from his or her perspective. Your presence in the classroom during the lesson will be tolerated better because the teacher and you have a shared understanding of what the lesson is about.

There is a transcript of a planning conference on pages 168–71.

Notes

1. Frances F. Fuller, "Concerns of Teachers: A Developmental Conceptualization," *American Educational Research Journal* 6 (1969): 207–26.
2. Ibid., 220–21.
3. Andrew J. Bush, John J. Kennedy, and Donald R. Cruikshank, "An Empirical Investigation of Teacher Clarity," *Journal of Teacher Education* 28 (1977): 53–58.
4. Mary L. Collins, "Effects of Enthusiasm Training on Preservice Elementary Teachers," *Journal of Teacher Education* 29 (1978): 53–57.

4

The Feedback Conference

"You're the first one around here who has helped me."
—Student comment

Several things must have taken place before a successful feedback conference can occur.

1. In a planning conference, teacher and supervisor have set some goals for the year, identified concerns, established a rationale for working together, considered the strategies the teacher has been using and intends to use, and translated abstract concerns into observable behaviors the supervisor can record.
2. Before an observation session, teacher and supervisor have identified the nature of the lesson, made the objectives explicit, discussed what the teacher will be doing (strategy), predicted what the students will be doing (expectations), considered specific problems or concerns the teacher anticipated in the observed lesson, and selected appropriate observation techniques or recording systems.
3. During the observational visit the supervisor has employed one or more devices from a repertoire of data recording techniques, has used appropriate recording devices for the specific situation as related to the goals and concerns, and has recorded data unobtrusively and without disruption of the class.

Now we are ready to begin a feedback conference.

The supervisor tries to provide objective observational data, analyze the data cooperatively and reach agreement with the teacher on what is happening. Then teacher and supervisor interpret the data. The supervisor elicits the teacher's reactions to the data (inferences, opinions, feelings) and considers possible causes and consequences. Together, teacher and supervisor reach decisions about future actions. These may be decisions about alternative teacher strategies, different objectives for students, or modification of the teacher's self-improvement goals. At this juncture, teacher and supervisor may recognize a need for other kinds of information or make plans for the next observation. Often, the feedback conference for one observation becomes the planning conference for the next.

Provide the Teacher with Feedback Using Objective Observational Data (Technique 22)

In one of our earliest workshops on observation and conference techniques, a principal remarked that making a chart of teacher movement seemed a strange thing to do. When given a chance to practice data gathering in an actual classroom, however, he tried a movement chart. He brought it back to the group, commenting on how much more *his* teacher had moved than had the teacher in our example. "And," he added, "the teacher looked at it afterward and said, 'This is really interesting information; you're the only principal who ever brought me something useful from an observation.' " The key to his unexpected success was that he had used the essential ingredient of effective conferences: providing objective data.

If the planning conference has established one or more goals that address genuine concerns and if the observational data are accurate and relevant, then the teacher should find the information useful, and the conference should run relatively smoothly. Many conferences are difficult because the data are "soft" (i.e., subjective, inaccurate, irrelevant). The inherent defensiveness teachers feel toward what they perceive as an evaluative situation is heightened by information that, to them, is suspect and debatable. "Hard" data alleviate this problem. Teachers do not say that what they saw on videotape or heard on audiotape did not happen, even though they may analyze or interpret events in a way that differs from the supervisor's analysis. Data in paper-and-pencil form (e.g., selected verbatim statements or seating charts) can be similarly convincing.

We should keep in mind, however, that all data are more or less subjective; even with videotape and film, someone chooses where to aim the camera and whether to take close-ups or long shots. Sound recordings can be affected by microphone placement and other factors. Checklists and charts are subject to the judgment, skill, and bias of the person tallying frequencies of given behaviors, choosing categories, or estimating qualitative ratings.

Similarly, in sharing information there is a temptation to add editorial opinion either through direct comment or through a not-so-subtle use of adjectives. Consider this statement: "Here are some objective unbiased data on your chaotic classroom."

Beginning the Conference

Having important information to discuss is the essential ingredient of a successful feedback conference. This means information that is objective (unbiased), accurate, clear (to both parties), relevant to the agreed-upon concerns, and interpretable in respect to what changes are feasible and reasonable. If the supervisor has this kind of information available in an easily displayed and readily understood form, a logical opening for the conference is "Let's look at the data we have collected."

Analyzing comes next, which means simply describing what the recorded information shows is happening without making value judgments. It is best for the teacher to take the lead in doing this.

Interpreting the data includes looking for probable causes of observed effects, or possible consequences, or suggested alternatives. Allowing the teacher to hypothesize several consequences or infer several reasonable causes of observed phenomena is usually a productive strategy. For example, repeated observations of student "at task" behaviors during a class period may show pupil interest in the activity waning after twenty minutes. The teacher may interpret this to indicate a weakness in the activity or a normal consequence of limited student attention span. Depending on the interpretation, decisions for change will vary. If the activity is judged inappropriate, it may be modified or changed substantially; if it is interpreted as appropriate but too long, it may merely need to be shortened.

Deciding what changes to make in future instruction can take many forms. Decisions can relate to any elements discussed in the planning conference. For example, the conferees may conclude that one or more of the following should be changed:

- The nature of the lesson or unit
- The objectives of the lesson or unit
- What the teacher does during the instruction
- What the students do during the instruction
- What additional kinds of information are needed to make intelligent decisions through analysis and interpretation

Another way of looking at decisions is to consider their magnitude. At one extreme, the teacher may decide to leave teaching as the result of systematic observational feedback (this has happened). At the other extreme, the teacher may decide not to change a thing (this has not happened, in our experience; teachers who believe they are perfect must be very rare). More often, teachers think of several aspects of the instruction that could be changed. The teacher may decide to experiment with these changes one at a time and analyze the effects. Usually the effects can be observed by the teacher without repeated visits by an observer, but in some cases an observer will be needed. In addition to the supervisor, other observers may be available— colleagues, aides, or even students.

Occasionally a teacher reaches a decision as the result of viewing data the supervisor provided without comments during the feedback conference. For example, a teacher may resolve to get rid of an annoying mannerism noted in watching a videotape or to spend more time working with a certain student after noting the student's behavior recorded on a seating chart observation record. One teacher, who was using a low-key style during a videotaped observation, displayed a dynamic style during the next observation (also videotaped). When asked by the supervisor about the obvious and abrupt change in teaching style, a matter that had not been mentioned in the previous conference, the teacher replied, "It wasn't until after I saw that first tape that I realized how undynamic I was. I swore I'd try something much different the next time!" Such a radical change is unusual, but this teacher found he was capable of a more energetic approach to teaching—at least occasionally.

Science makes use of accurate data to understand, predict, and thereby control. Similarly, when presented with factual information rather than inferential conclusions drawn by the supervisor, the teacher is in a position to behave professionally and responsibly in the next step.

Elicit the Teacher's Inferences, Opinions, and Feelings (Technique 23)

Providing objective data (technique 21) can be translated into practice as, "Here's what I recorded from your lesson; let's have a look at it." The technique we are about to discuss, eliciting reactions, does *not* call for an opening question like, "How do you feel your lesson went?" Cautious teachers hesitate to say, "Great!" for fear you will contradict or disagree. On the other hand, if they say, "Lousy," they run the risk of having you agree. "Some parts were good, others could be improved" is a safe answer, but this is what the conference is all about anyway. The supervisor can choose a less threatening opener, after the teacher has had a chance to inspect the information, by asking, "What aspects of the data do you want to talk about first?"

Eliciting the teacher's reactions to the data requires skill and patience. There is always a temptation to jump to conclusions about what has been observed and recorded before the teacher has had an opportunity to reflect on it. A device that works well, especially in connection with tape recordings, is to ask the following questions:

"What do you see [or hear] in the record [or tape] that you would repeat if you did this lesson again?"

"What would you change?"

"If you were a student in the class, what would you want to change?"

We have asked these questions of hundreds of teachers—primary, intermediate, secondary, and college teachers—who have viewed videotapes of themselves. No one has answered all the questions with "I wouldn't change a thing." If "What would you repeat?" gets no response, you can proceed immediately to the second question. If the teacher expresses total satisfaction with the lesson in response to "What would you change?" the third question, "What would a student want changed?" should provoke a more thoughtful response. The teacher can be asked to view the instruction from the perspective of different students, say, one who usually has difficulty understanding and one who is usually ahead of the rest.

These questions are phrased in a relatively nonthreatening manner to which most teachers are able to respond openly and with considerable insight. In response to the third question, one teacher said,

T: "Which student?"

S: "What do you mean, which student?"

T: "Well, the slowest, the brightest, the least interested?"

S: OK, the slowest."

T: "All right. What I see that teacher doing is talking too fast, using vocabulary I don't understand, discussing topics that don't affect me. I don't think she likes me; she never calls on me even when I know the answer."

This was a healthy insight for the teacher to develop, and the anecdote points out that one function of the supervisor is to serve as a catalyst, to help the teacher make productive use of the available information.

For most teachers, the steps in the feedback conference are reasonable and appropriate: providing objective data, analyzing and interpreting it, and drawing conclusions with the teacher taking equal part in a collaborative process. Unfortunately, many supervisors reverse the process. They provide their own conclusions, give some analysis that justifies the conclusions, then search for data to substantiate the analysis. Often, no alternative interpretations are even considered.

For a small percentage of teachers a "conclusions first" conference approach may be needed. For example, it may be more effective to say, "You've been late for work twelve times this month. This has got to stop, or else!" rather than to say, "Here are some data about your punctuality. Do you find anything of interest?" An alternative effective strategy could be "What do you propose to do about this record of tardiness?"

There are several assumptions in a procedure that encourages teachers to come to their own conclusions, based on objective information and thoughtful analysis:

- Few teachers set out deliberately to do a bad job. Most have reasonable goals.
- Most teachers have alternative strategies available and can use them if they see a need.
- We don't "see ourselves as others see us." Being able to view our teaching from a new perspective can be an enlightening experience.
- Those insights we discover for ourselves tend to be retained and acted on with more energy and better spirit than those we are told about by others.
- Many teachers prefer a collaborative, collegial approach instead of one in which the supervisor is regarded as "superior."
- Good data can be more persuasive than mere admonishments.

Persuasive data contain no value judgments. Inferences and generalizations the *observer* may have formed about the activity are not included in the data presented in a conference with the teacher. Data
that might lead the teacher to the same inferences probably should be
presented, however. Persuasive data, in addition to being value-free,
must be specific and presented in a form that can be understood and
used immediately by the teacher. They also must be data the teacher
feels are necessary and important at a given time. For example, a
teacher concerned about the inability to ask good questions is probably not ready for data and conferences designed to improve lecturing prowess. Or data that might be helpful to a teacher worried
about disciplinary problems might be regarded as irrelevant by a
teacher who has no problem with discipline. The observer needs a
variety of skills to share data in a persuasive manner at a time when
the teacher feels that the data are relevant, important, and useful.

One elementary teacher, after studying a seating chart on which an
observer had recorded which students were responded to by the
teacher (and in what ways), began to understand why some students
felt "turned off" and planned activities that created opportunities to
respond in positive ways to those students. Many teachers who have
analyzed charts of their direct and indirect behaviors (using Flanders's categories) have modified the indirect-direct ratio. Teachers
who have had access to verbal flow patterns on seating charts (who
talks to whom) often have been stimulated to experiment with different seating arrangements.

A high school science teacher studied observational charts that
showed what percent of his students were "at task" for various
time periods. The percentages were strikingly high, which might
have been expected to please this instructor. Yet the teacher concluded that they were "too high." Every year a number of students
dropped this course; after the instructor saw the data, he realized he
was "keeping their noses to the grindstone" so much that the course
was unduly punishing. He decided to restructure the course.

When a supervisor feels that a teacher is drawing acceptable inferences and suggesting reasonable alternative plans for the future a
simple reinforcement is all the technique needed. The supervisor can
say, "That sounds like a good idea, Pat. Why don't you try it?"

Another teacher had been having some real problems with lesson
preparation and control of students. She was observed on two successive days, the observer taking verbatim notes of her questions and
control statements. At the feedback conference, the observer began
the conference as follows:

S: "How do you feel about the two lessons?"

T: "Well, I feel that it went better today than yesterday. But how did I look?"

S: "You know I'm not going to answer that."

T: "I know."

It would have been better for the observer to start the dialogue with

S: "Here are the questions and control statements you wanted to analyze. Let's have a look at them."

If the teacher asks "How did I do?" an appropriate answer is "Let's see." Then teacher and supervisor turn to the data.

Encourage the Teacher to Consider Alternative Lesson Objectives, Methods, Reasons (Technique 24)

Once a supervisor has analyzed the data, the tendency is to say to a teacher, "Here's what I would do if I were you." This short-circuits the system. If teaching were a straightforward physical skill, then viewing the performance and giving advice like "Keep your eye on the ball" would be effective. Translated to advice about teaching this tends to become "Be firm, fair, and consistent." This is undoubtedly good advice, but it does not tell what to be firm about (discipline? standards? questionable rules? teacher opinions?) or what is fair and consistent for all (activities for the physically handicapped? individualized academic assignments?). Moreover, there are always feasible alternatives for teaching anything. When change is desired, one purpose of the feedback conference is to get the teacher to consider several alternatives and choose the most promising. Teachers should be able to give alternative explanations of why things might be happening the way they are and also to suggest several ways to change the situation, or the strategy, or the activities.

Student teachers and beginning teachers have a more limited repertoire of possible approaches than do more experienced teachers. One benefit accruing from systematic observation and teacher-centered conferences should be teachers who, on their own volition, do self-analyses using objective data and thus develop a wider range of alternative approaches.

For example, a group of beginning teachers in an intern program read about social-class discrimination by teachers in schools. They recorded their own interactions with students in their classes, played them back, and were surprised to learn that they, too, were favoring middle-class children.

Another group of inexperienced teachers asked for help in learning how to control student participation in recitations and discussions. They were asked to note several students who were often active participants in a lesson and several others who seldom participated. In the next lesson they were asked to see if they could limit those who talked the most to no more than three contributions and get those who rarely participated to make at least three contributions. Every teacher reported being able to accomplish this assignment without any special instructions; simply being aware of the two groups of students was all that was necessary.

Many aspects of teaching can be observed, recorded, and analyzed as easily as counting student contributions to a recitation or discussion. You may wonder why teachers are not more aware of such obvious patterns as paying more attention to one side of the room or calling only on students in the front seats. The answer is that these things are not obvious to teachers while they are preoccupied with the details of teaching. They are not obvious to observers either, unless they are watching for them.

Supervisors often feel that if they record specific information, such as the nature of the teacher's responses to individual students, they will miss other important elements of the teaching-learning situation. Our experience suggests that we see more as observers when we have something specific on which to focus our attention. Making an audiotape recording in addition to whatever charts or codes the observer is keeping on paper ensures back-up information about the lesson if it is needed.

A common worry among beginning teachers is the problem of discipline. Students can get out of hand whether they are first graders or high school seniors. Feedback on this aspect of teaching can bring startling results. One of our practice teachers asked that we videotape her troublesome fifth-period class instead of the well-behaved first-period class we had taped twice before. She volunteered the tape for analysis in a seminar on a day when classroom discipline was to be discussed and a film was to be shown that illustrated both ineffective and effective techniques. When her classroom tape was played later in the session, the teacher was able to see herself using many of the ineffective techniques portrayed in the film.

Provide the Teacher with Opportunities for Practice and Comparison (Technique 25)

As a source of alternative teaching methods, a supervisor may be asked to play a more direct role as a model for a teacher by demonstrating a particular method or technique in the classroom. Curriculum specialists in particular are often asked to do such demonstrations. When this is done, the teacher becomes the observer and records data to be analyzed and interpreted in a postdemonstration conference. For example, an elementary teacher was experiencing difficulty explaining "pi" and the formulas $C = \pi d$ and $A = \pi r^2$. She asked a mathematics specialist to take over a lesson while she observed the explanation and recorded student questions. During the feedback conference, information about the supervisor's lesson was incorporated into information taken from the teacher's experience and plans.

Another frequent strategy is to suggest that one teacher observe another in order to compare styles or strategies or pick up some different techniques. If the observing teacher has some knowledge of systematic observation and recording, the feedback conference can result in a mutual sharing of ideas and perspectives.

Time for collecting information and providing feedback is always limited. Most supervisors should spend more time on these activities than they typically do; even those supervisors who allot the most time feel a need for more. One way to increase the amount of feedback is for the teacher to collect some of it. This can be done with teacher-made tape recordings (audio or video), by getting systematic feedback from students or by using teacher aides or colleagues as observers.

When data come from sources other than the supervisor's observations and are analyzed by the teacher without a structured conference, some guidelines are needed. The supervisor can help the teacher pick a central focus for the self-analysis. This can be one of the goals for the year that the teacher and the supervisor set at the first planning conference. Or it can be a concentration on a certain technique the teacher wishes to strengthen, say, asking better questions or moderating group discussions, giving clearer explanations and directions, or exhibiting more warmth and enthusiasm.

Care needs to be taken in selecting an appropriate source of information. For topics like those in the preceding paragraph, audiotape recordings would be reasonable. Information about how instruction is being individualized might come from an adult observer or from the students themselves. Several instruments are available for collecting student feedback. The products of student work also can be analyzed in relation to the teacher's goals.

The teacher can incorporate self-analysis activities in a future feedback conference. For example, one teacher discovered a surprising and unsuspected number of "put-downs" in his informal interactions with students. He was determined to make several ten- or fifteen-minute tape recordings each week at times when he would be interacting informally with groups. The supervisor suggested that the teacher note the frequency of such remarks in the samples over time and write examples of what he had said along with alternative phrases he could have used. The next time teacher and supervisor got together, both were pleased with the progress that had been made. Moreover, they agreed it would be useful for the supervisor to check the perceptions of a few students informally.

Beginning teachers need systematic practice in using a variety of strategies and techniques. Many of these can be practiced without direct supervision and recorded for self-analysis. Here are some common strategies along with suggested means of "self-observation."

Strategy	Self-Observational Device
Lecture: explanations, directions	Audiotape recording, selective verbatim*
Discussion, seminar	Verbal flow chart* made by student or by teacher using tape recording
Demonstration	Videotape recording
Individualized instruction: seatwork, resource centers, laboratory, shop	Classroom traffic (movement) chart* drawn by aide
Simulations, games, self-instructional materials	"At task" chart* prepared by teacher as students participate
Heuristic approaches: problem solving, inquiry lessons, guided discovery.	Selective verbatim of teacher questions or student questions taken from tape recording

*These devices are described in the next section.

If the teacher has collected and analyzed some of the data, much time can be saved in a subsequent conference with the supervisor. Some tasks the teacher can perform also will make the teacher better-informed at the time of the conference. For example, transcribing selected verbatim from a tape, charting student participation, or plotting frequencies from a student questionnaire will make the teacher aware of elements that need improvement or emphasis.

The feedback conference can also be shortened if the supervisor provides the teacher ahead of time with the data that will be discussed. It is often convenient to make a carbon or NCR copy when data is being recorded. After the lesson, the observer can say to the teacher, "Here's a copy of the raw data. Look it over before we meet, and I'll do the same."

Summary

In this chapter we have described the techniques essential to a clinical supervision feedback conference:

(1) Provide the teacher with feedback using objective observational data. If the data are inadequate, inaccurate, biased, or irrelevant to the teacher's concerns, the process cannot get started. The teacher must feel that the information being analyzed is a valid representation of what is really happening in the classroom. Information that relies on memory is less persuasive than information that is objectively recorded.

(2) Elicit the teacher's inferences, opinions, and feelings about the observational data. If the data are accurate and objective, but the supervisor immediately draws opinionated inferences from the data, the teacher may feel compelled to respond defensively rather than interpret the data in a self-directed and productive way. It takes self-control and practice to provide another person with data in a nonevaluative, nonthreatening manner. The use of adjectives or nonverbal cues may communicate opinions or conclusions to the teacher before he or she has had a chance to work through the steps.

(3) Encourage the teacher to consider alternative lesson objectives, methods, reasons. If the teacher expresses dissatisfaction with something observed in the lesson, several reasonable hypotheses may help explain why an event is occurring; it is a mistake to zero in on only one possibility. Similarly, several feasible alternatives are usually available for dealing with a problem; more than one should be considered before settling on the best alternative. Here the supervisor can help the teacher avoid two traps: (1) "functional fixedness," proceeding to judge all information on the basis of a single hypothesis (which may

be wrong); and (2) "a working definition of insanity," considering only one solution to a problem and when that doesn't work, doubling and redoubling our efforts with the same unsuccessful approach. The collaborative setting of the conference should provide teacher and supervisor with a wider range of hypotheses and proposed solutions than either conferee could generate alone.

Ⓐ *Provide the teacher with opportunities for practice and comparison*. Because the teacher has settled on a plan of action, the supervisor should not expect to see the problem solved immediately. Teachers need time to try out new approaches, develop new skills, or compare several strategies. The supervisor can follow up at a later time to observe, record, and reinforce teacher progress.

Ideally, the feedback conference takes the following form:

1. The observer *displays the data* recorded during the observation. This is done without evaluative comments.
2. The teacher *analyzes* what was happening during the lesson as evidenced by the data. The supervisor simply helps to clarify what behaviors the recorded data represent.
3. The teacher, with the help of the supervisor, *interprets* the behaviors of teacher and students as represented by the observational data. At this stage the teacher becomes more evaluative because causes and consequences must be discussed as desirable or undesirable.
4. The teacher, with assistance (sometimes guidance) from the supervisor, *decides* on alternative approaches for the future to attend to dissatisfactions with the observed teaching or to emphasize those aspects that were satisfying.
5. The supervisor *reinforces* the teacher's announced intentions for change when the supervisor agrees with them or helps the teacher modify the intentions if there is some disagreement.

Supervisors are often surprised at how easily these steps can be accomplished. When supplied with adequate information and allowed to act on it, most teachers can analyze, interpret, and decide in a self-directed and constructive manner. When things do not go well in a feedback conference, the difficulties can usually be traced to failure on the part of the supervisor to use an effective clinical supervision technique.

There is a transcript of a feedback conference on page 174–79.

5

Direct and Indirect Styles of Supervision

"Take my advice: don't give advice."—Anonymous

The techniques in chapter 4 can be used by any supervisor who has systematically collected observational data to analyze with a teacher. How the data are interpreted and what decisions are reached will depend to a considerable extent on the supervisor's style. Styles of supervision can be described in many ways; we shall use a common distinction: direct versus indirect styles.

Flanders[1] differentiates direct teaching styles (i.e., lecturing, directing, criticizing) from indirect styles (i.e., accepting feelings, encouraging, acknowledging, using student ideas). Blumberg[2] uses similar categories for supervisor behavior and has gathered some evidence that teachers prefer an indirect sytle of supervision.

The direct and indirect behaviors a supervisor may employ can be placed on a continuum, though no scale is intended.

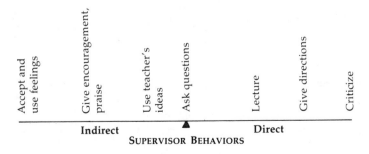

| Accept and use feelings | Give encouragement, praise | Use teacher's ideas | Ask questions | Lecture | Give directions | Criticize |

Indirect ▲ Direct

SUPERVISOR BEHAVIORS

Another range of possible conference behaviors on the teacher's part can be constructed using the work of Spaulding.[3]

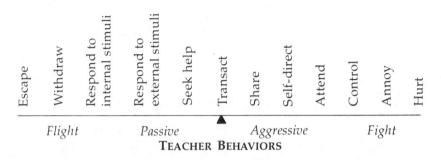

Escape	Withdraw	Respond to internal stimuli	Respond to external stimuli	Seek help	Transact	Share	Self-direct	Attend	Control	Annoy	Hurt

Flight   *Passive*   ▲   *Aggressive*   *Fight*

TEACHER BEHAVIORS

The behavior of either conferee can be described with labels used by Shostrom.[4]

Warm	Sensitive	Dependent	Supportive	Controlling	Critical	Strong	Aggressive

CHARACTERISTICS OF CONFEREES

These characteristics can be translated into verbs that describe a range of verbal behavior the supervisor or teacher can employ.

Care	Guide	Appreciate	Empathize	Respect	Express	Lead	Assert

One can also view the supervisor's actions as aversive (dominative, punishing) or supportive (approving, receptive). Setting limits and setting goals are actions that usually lie between these extremes but can be pushed toward one end or the other.

Approving Receptive Setting Goals Setting Limits Dominating Punishing

Supportive   *Aversive*

Although teachers indicate a preference for supervisors who emphasize the supportive, caring style, these are not the only appropriate behaviors for a supervisor. A caring style at times may be indicated by doing something aversive (e.g., when a parent prevents a child from playing on the highway).

This chapter recommends several techniques usually regarded as indirect, but they also can be used by direct supervisors. Indeed they should be so used when persuasive data are shared. The techniques are concerned with listening, acknowledging, clarifying, encouraging, guiding (rather than directing), supporting, and dealing with feelings.

The techniques that follow are especially useful for supervisors who want conferences to be "teacher-centered." Whether a supervisor's essential style is direct or indirect, self-centered or teacher-centered, these techniques can be used to improve the quality of interaction between the conferees.

Listen More, Talk Less (Technique 26)

Many supervisors dominate the conversation. The teacher has little chance to identify goals and objectives, analyze and interpret information, or reach decisions about future actions. Teachers talk to students about two thirds of the time they teach, and supervisors talk in about the same proportion to teachers. The exact ratio varies, but too many supervisors do most of the talking. It is difficult to attend to a teacher's concerns in a conference or encourage a teacher's plans for improvement when the supervisor monopolizes the conference. Avoid this tendency when applying the techniques in the remainder of this chapter.

Acknowledge, Paraphrase, and Use What the Teacher Is Saying (Technique 27)

Supervisors who insert an "I understand" or "I know what you mean" in the course of a teacher's conversation indicate that they are listening. Accurate paraphrases also show that they understand the teacher. Using the teacher's ideas can be even more convincing than merely acknowledging (hearing) or paraphrasing (comprehending) them. Applying an idea to a different situation is but one example; pointing to a logical consequence is another. Paraphrasing can be overdone if too many responses are similar, or if they are inappropriately placed. For example, if a teacher says, "The car was going sixty miles an hour," it doesn't contribute much to respond, "What you are saying is that the automobile was traveling a mile a minute." An effective paraphrase must be a genuine effort to communicate that we understand what the other person is getting at. Using an idea of the teacher's shows that the supervisor heard, understood and is pursuing the thought. Of course, it can be pursued so far that it ceases to be the teacher's idea and becomes the supervisor's. Generally, however, having a person you respect use your idea is rewarding.

Ask Clarifying Questions (Technique 28)

The teacher's statements often need to be probed to clarify the supervisor's understanding and to get the teacher to think carefully about inferences and decisions. "Tell me what you mean by that" or "Can you say a little more about that?" are examples. So are "What would you accept as evidence that _____ is happening?" "Do you know someone who is especially good at that? What does he do?" "Would you give me a specific example?"

In many instances, if we do not clarify, miscommunication is the result. Occasionally someone will say, "You're absolutely right! Moreover, . . ." And then the person proceeds to say the exact opposite of what you thought you said. Of course, that also could be a conscious strategy or a case of not listening at all, but a clarifying question avoids unintentional misunderstandings.

An example of paraphrasing and asking clarifying questions took place in a high school where the principal gave the faculty an administrator appraisal form to fill out anonymously. After analyzing the compiled responses, the principal said in a faculty meeting, "What you seem to be telling me in this survey is that I'm not as accessible as you would like." Several teachers said, almost in unison, "Could you tell us what 'being accessible' would look like?" To which the principal replied: "Well, I'd keep my door open more and welcome 'drop-in' chats. And if you stopped me in the hall and asked a question, I'd try to answer it briefly instead of pointing out that I was on my way to a meeting."

Having announced and clarified his intentions in public, he was destined to become "Mr. Accessible" in the next few months. Of course he had some help from wags on the faculty who could not resist asking, "Are you feeling accessible?"

Several points can be made with this example: (1) the paraphrase translated a statistic into flesh-and-blood behavior, (2) the clarifying question checked the perceptions of the subject and his observers, and (3) the public announcement of a resolution to change virtually ensured success. The same process takes place in the feedback conference. Note that the principal had objective data, analyzed and interpreted the data, made a decision, made use of paraphrasing and clarifying questions, and received verbal support in his resolve to change. These are exactly the steps we should follow in helping teachers improve their teaching.

Give Specific Praise for Teacher Performance and Growth (Technique 29)

To say "That was a nice lesson" is not specific praise. Saying "That was an excellent answer you gave to Billy" or "Removing Fred from the group was an effective way to handle the problem" makes the approval explicit. It is especially important to note positive instances where the teacher has shown growth toward an avowed goal.

There is some possibility that a supervisor will reinforce more than was bargained for. A workshop leader received this comment from a participant on the postworkshop evaluation: "Stopping the tape recording to explain what was happening was really helpful." So the leader stopped the tape about twenty times during the next workshop, until someone sent this note: "Why don't you let the tape play long enough for us to hear what's going on?"

Again, an elderly lady who had never eaten apple pie remarked that when she was a girl, she turned down her first opportunity to do so and gained considerable attention: "Imagine that! Carrie doesn't eat apple pie." The attention was such that in subsequent situations, she felt compelled to continue her refusal, although she confessed, "I always thought I might have liked it."

Yet in our experience, the possibility of too little reinforcement for teachers is much more likely than too much. Teaching often seems a thankless task to those who toil in the schools of our nation. They seldom lack critics, however.

Avoid Giving Direct Advice (Technique 30)

This does not say *never* give direct advice, just wait a while. Let teachers analyze and interpret. Often the decisions they reach will be very similar to yours. For most teachers, having their ideas for change reinforced by someone they respect is more likely to produce results than having to carry out someone else's idea. On the other hand, there are times when it is better to say what we think rather than let indirectness become manipulative.

Some people are naturally compliant, submissive, obedient;

perhaps they enjoy being told what to do. Nevertheless, our experience with teachers indicates that most of them prefer to feel responsible for their own actions. People who choose teaching as a career expect to be in charge of their classes; they expect to make professional decisions about goals, subject matter, materials, methodology, evaluation, and other aspects of the educational process.

The line between "guided discovery" and "manipulation" is a fine one. The supervisor must decide when "Here's the way it looks to me" is preferable to making the teacher feel that guessing games are being played.

Provide Verbal Support (Technique 31)

The emphasis of the supervisor is on helping the teacher identify professional goals relating to classroom performance, then obtaining valid feedback to assist in reaching those goals. It is often difficult for teachers to separate personal goals from professional goals, and it is especially difficult to separate personal problems from professional ones. Many of the problems administrators identify as deterrents to instructional improvement by their teachers have their basis in personal aspects of the teacher's life—for example, apathy, lack of organization, or emotional instability in the classroom.

It would be convenient if we could exclude personal problems from a discussion of techniques to use in conducting conferences, yet they often enter the discussion despite all efforts to stay on a professional level. Most supervisors have had the experience of a teacher crying at some point in a conference. Analyzing behavior is an intensely personal process that often defies a scientific or cold-blooded approach.

Hence, we need ways of dealing with these situations as they arise. It does not seem reasonable for the supervisor to be in tears along with the teacher, yet some expression of sympathy or empathy is in order. If the problems seem to be medical or psychiatric, the course of action is clear: seek help by referring the teacher to an appropriate specialist. Teacher supervisors and school administrators are not competent to make medical diagnoses ("He's an alcoholic" or "She's mentally ill"), and it is definitely not advisable to attempt psychiatric therapy or psychological counseling without the necessary special training and experience. On the other hand, if the problem does not seem to require professional, medical, or psychiatic treatment, a sympathetic listener can often help a person work through a problem.

At the beginning of chapter 4 there is a statement from a university student: "You're the first one around here who has helped me!" This student had sought aid from several advisers in solving a personal problem. One faculty member took the time to listen to the particulars then said, "It seems to me you've identified several possible alternatives. You could drop out of school and work full-time for a while, or you could take a reduced load and work part-time; and you also need to decide whether to get married now or wait." With his own alternatives outlined, the student said, "I see now what I need to do. Thank you."

Client-centered counseling doesn't always work out as quickly or as well, but for a number of reasons it may be an appropriate strategy for the supervisory conference with a teacher. The supervisor does not necessarily know more about teaching kindergarten, French, or physics than the teacher; is probably not aware of as many factors in this particular classroom situation as the teacher; does not expect to spend the rest of the term, year, or career in this teacher's classroom; and will probably rely on the teacher to do most of the follow-up on decisions. It is within the domain of the supervisor to consider what the teacher says about personal problems in the light of how they pertain to performance in the classroom.

The level of trust the two people have established is a major variable in how helpful a supervisor can be to a teacher with a personal problem that may be interfering with classroom effectiveness. Several factors influence trust building. We tend to trust those who trust us. We tend to trust those whose competence we respect. One way to build a teacher's confidence in our competence as supervisors is to demonstrate our ability to provide useful feedback and to conduct productive conferences.

In some cases a supervisor needs to take full charge of the dealings with certain teachers: selecting what kinds of data will be collected and then analyzing and interpreting that information, drawing conclusions about which goals are being met and which are not, and deciding what needs to be done in the future. At the other extreme, a supervisor may encourage some teachers to set their own goals, select appropriate information to use in assessing the achievement of those goals, and make decisions about future efforts. As pedagogical strategies, these approaches are either didactic or heuristic. How much structure supervisors provide for a conference will depend on their estimate of what kind of atmosphere will provide maximum potential for the growth of a particular teacher.

We have found that when teachers are given a choice of supervisors, some choose one they know to be quite direct whereas others prefer one who tends to be indirect. Teachers who prefer the direct approach may say "I know where she stands" or "He tells it like it is" or "I'm tired of people 'bouncing everything off the wall.' " Those who like an indirect style may say "I feel more comfortable with Mary; she doesn't act like she has all the answers" or "Fred helps me do my own thinking and treats me like a colleague" or "I've had enough of the 'hardsell' approach."

The classroom observer is often cast in a double role: as a colleague helping to improve instruction and as an evaluator. It is sometimes awkward to deal with these two functions simultaneously. For example, to say "I'll devote the first few visits to helping you improve and save the evaluating until later" does not reassure the teacher, nor can the observer forget what has been seen. With teachers who are doing reasonably well, this need not be a problem: "I'm expecting to write a favorable evaluation anyway, so let's concentrate on some areas you'd like to work on" is one approach. Teachers on the borderline deserve to be informed of this fact, but the conferences can still be positive and productive. Fair dismissal procedures also require that teachers be given early notice of deficiencies and assistance in attempting to overcome them.

In a few cases, the teacher may be in an "intensive evaluation" situation. (Some districts encourage such a teacher to have an attorney or teachers' organization representative in attendance at any conferences with an evaluator.) Obviously, the tone of the conference will be different in the intensive case. Yet supervisors do not have to turn from Jekyll into Hyde. A skillful parent serves as both counselor and disciplinarian and can do so in a consistent style. Supervisors, too, should be able to fulfill both aspects of their role skillfully.

Dissonance theory provides a rationale for changing teachers' classroom behavior through observational feedback and teacher-centered conferences. The writings of Festinger,[5] Heider,[6] and others supply powerful insights into the dynamics of what Burns expressed in poetic form as the gift of seeing ourselves as others see us. We each have an externally perceived self and an internally perceived self. We develop discomfort when we become aware of a discrepancy between what we believe to be "the real me" and what "the perceived me" seems to be doing—in the eyes of others or in the information collected through systematic observation. For example, a teacher who believes that teachers should smile a lot feels that he smiles a lot; if he views videotapes of himself that show no smiles, he has dissonance. This dissonance can be reduced in several ways, such as:

1. "The videotape is wrong."
2. "It was a bad day, I was nervous."
3. "It isn't really that important to smile so often."

In other words, he can (1) deny the information, (2) reduce the importance of the information, or (3) reduce the importance of the behavior. Another possibility is that he can resolve to make the perceived self more like the "real" or ideal self. That requires changing his behavior.

The goal of supervision for instructional improvement is to get teachers to change their behavior in ways that both they and their supervisors regard as desirable. In some cases only the supervisor (and not the teacher) sees a suggested change as desirable. Now the supervisor experiences dissonance. Among the options for reducing this dissonance are

1. "You'll do it my way, or I'll send you to Siberia."
2. "Let's look at some more data about what is happening."
3. "Let's work on something *you* are concerned about."

In other words, the supervisor may (1) reduce dissonance by forcing compliance from the teacher or (2) and (3) attempt to achieve consonance through increased understanding of what is in the teacher's mind.

There are times when it is necessary to force teacher compliance to the supervisor's demands—for example, when laws or official school policies are at stake. Most problems that supervisors and teachers work on are not that clear-cut. They concern ways of dealing with students; choosing strategies for teaching certain concepts, skills, or facts; finding alternative ways of managing the many variables in teaching; selecting elements of teaching style that can be modified by the teacher through the use of feedback, practice, and experimentation.

It is unlikely that a teacher can alter a fundamental personality characteristic like dominance, emotional stability, or empathy. Nevertheless, a teacher can learn to use strategies that reduce the tendency to dominate or can develop classroom management techniques that reduce emotional stress. Some outward and visible signs of empathy can be observed, practiced, and incorporated into a teacher's repertoire without resorting to psychiatric therapy or profound religious conversion. Most people who choose teaching as a career have basic qualities that are compatible with the requirements of the job; systematic feedback can inform and convince those who do not.

Acknowledge and Use What the Person Is Feeling (Technique 32)

Rogers[7] reminds us that when a child attempts to do something difficult and says, "I can't," a typical parental response is, "Of course you can!" The response is intended to be positive, but it denies feelings. It might not hurt to say, "It *is* difficult, isn't it, but you'll get it."

Researchers have found that feelings are seldom acknowledged verbally in the classroom.[8] The occurrence in conferences is less well documented, but we suspect that it is unduly limited. When the goal is to change behavior, affective aspects cannot be ignored. The emotions that can be expressed in a conference range from rage to despair, from exhilaration to depression. Clinical supervisors should not ignore the significant emotional content of what teachers are saying any more than they would ignore important cognitive statements.

One way to respond is to describe what you are observing: "You appear to be quite angry about that" or "This seems to make you anxious." Don't be surprised if the teacher's response is "Oh, no, I'm not really angry" or "Who's anxious? I'm not anxious." We tend to deny feelings, as if it were bad to have them, especially in a teaching situation. A psychologist once remarked, "I always knew when my mother was angry at me because she showed it immediately, and I could take that; but my father would wait to 'have a talk with me later,' and that was an agonizing experience." Expressing feelings can be healthy and helpful.

After an expecially satisfying performance before a large class of graduate students, the instructor was told by one student, "I enjoyed seeing that you were relishing the experience." That is a good observation to share. Telling a teacher "You appeared to be enjoying the responses you were getting" or "I shared your apprehension when Dickie volunteered" can have a desirable effect on the tone of the discussion.

Counseling

For many years we advised supervisors to avoid taking on a counseling role with teachers. We thought it best for supervisors to spend what time they had helping teachers improve their instructional efforts rather than attempting to work on marital, financial, or psychological problems. We felt that the "amateur psychiatrist" would do more harm than good. In the case of serious problems, we still feel this way, but we have modified our position somewhat.

The more we work with supervisors, the more we recognize that it is impossible for them to separate teachers' instructional problems from their personal problems. What is needed is an approach that avoids the pitfalls of inept amateur therapy yet deals honestly with problems expressed by the teacher that have significant impact on classroom performance.

For example, if a teacher says, "I'm spending so much time fighting with my spouse that I just can't get my lessons prepared," the supervisor might do one of several things:

- Threaten to fire the teacher if work does not improve
- Offer advice on how to improve a marriage
- Concentrate on ways of handling schoolwork at school
- Recommend a counselor
- Provide nondirective counseling

Any of the above might work, depending on the situation and the nature of the individuals involved. An objective approach consistent with other techniques in this chapter might be the following:

Supervisor: "Here are some of the things you've mentioned that would be desirable. Let's indicate them briefly in one column. Here are some things you have identified about the current situation. Let's put them in another column. Now you can add or subtract from either list, but the essential problem is to ask what it takes to get from here to there."

It is conceivable that a conscientious supervisor might perform all the tasks of planning, observing, and giving feedback (as recorded and coded by reliable means) and still not be regarded as helpful by the teacher. We suspect that when this happens, other personality factors or interpersonal dynamics account for the discrepancy. The data we have on what teachers want from a supervisor suggest a fairly open and democratic approach for most teachers. Yet we can use open and democratic procedures to communicate content that is quite structured. Discovery—guided discovery—and didactic teaching are examples of procedures that lie along this continuum.

Rogers,[9] who pioneered client-centered counseling in the 1940s, argues in a recent book for "person-centered" approaches in a wide range of human activities. He contrasts our usual notions of power and control with another view of influence and impact.

Some Notes on Leadership: Two Extremes

Influence and Impact	Power and Control
Giving autonomy to persons and groups	Making decisions
Freeing people to "do their thing"	Giving orders
Expressing own ideas and feelings as one aspect of the group data	Directing subordinates' behavior
Facilitating learning	Keeping own ideas and feelings "close to the vest"
Stimulating independence in thought and action	Exercising authority over people and organization
Accepting the "unacceptable" innovative creations that emerge	Dominating when necessary Coercing when necessary
Delegating, giving full responsibility	Teaching, instructing, advising
Offering feedback and receiving it	
Encouraging and relying on self-evaluation	Evaluating others
Finding rewards in the development and achievements of others	Giving rewards; being rewarded by own achievements

For most teachers, influence and impact are needed from supervisors, not power and control.

Management

Douglas McGregor's *The Human Side of Enterprise*[10] suggests two approaches to management, theory X and theory Y. They are not opposite poles on a continuum but two different views about work—including teaching and supervising. Theory X applies to traditional management and the assumptions underlying it. Theory Y is based on assumptions derived from research in the social sciences.

Three basic assumptions of theory X are these:

1. The average human being has an inherent dislike of work and will avoid it if possible.

2. Because of this human dislike of work, most people must be coerced, directed, and threatened with punishment to get them to put forth adequate effort toward the achievement of organizational objectives.
3. The average human being prefers to be directed, wishes to avoid responsibility, has relatively little ambition and wants security above all.

McGregor indicates that the "carrot and the stick" theory of motivation fits reasonably well with theory X. External rewards and punishments are the motivators of workers. The consequent direction and control does not recognize intrinsic human motivation.

Theory Y is more humanistic and is based on six assumptions:

1. The expenditure of physical and mental effort in work is as natural as play or rest.
2. External controls and the threat of punishment are not the only means for bringing about effort toward organizational objectives. Human beings will exercise self-direction and self-control in the service of objectives to which they are committed.
3. Commitment to objectives is a function of the rewards associated with their achievement.
4. The average human being learns, under proper conditions, not only to accept but also to seek responsibility.
5. The capacity to exercise a relatively high degree of imagination, ingenuity, and creativity in the solution of organizational problems is widely, not narrowly, distributed in the population.
6. Under the conditions of modern industrial life, the intellectual potentialities of the average human being are only partially utilized.

McGregor saw these assumptions leading to superior-subordinate relationships in which the subordinate would have greater influence over the activities in his or her own work and also have influence on the superior's actions. Through participatory management, greater creativity and productivity are expected, and also a greater sense of personal accomplishment and satisfaction by the workers. Argyris,[11] Bennis,[12] and Likert[13] cite evidence that a participatory system of management can be more effective than traditional management.

Likert's studies showed that high production can be achieved by managers oriented toward people rather than production. Moreover, these high-production managers were willing to delegate; to allow subordinates to participate in decisions; to be relatively nonpunitive;

and to use open, two-way communication patterns. High morale and effective planning were also characteristic of these "person-centered" managers. The results may be applied to the supervisory relationship in education as well as to industry.

Notes

1. Edmund Amidon and Ned Flanders, "Interaction Analysis as a Feedback System," *Interaction Analysis: Theory, Research, and Application,* ed. Edmund Amidon and John Hough, (Reading, MA: Addison-Wesley, 1967), pp. 122–124.
2. Arthur Blumberg, *Supervisors and Teachers: A Private Cold War* (Berkeley, CA: McCutchan, 1974).
3. Robert L. Spaulding, *A Coping Analysis Schedule for Educational Settings (CASES),* in *Mirrors for Behavior,* ed. Anita Simon and E. Gil Boyer, (Philadelphia: Research for Better Schools, 1967).
4. Everett L. Shostrom, *Man, the Manipulator* (Nashville, TN: Abingdon, 1967).
5. Leon Festinger, *A Theory of Cognitive Dissonance* (Stanford, CA: Stanford University Press, 1968).
6. Fritz Heider, *The Psychology of Interpersonal Relations* (New York: Wiley, 1958).
7. Carl R. Rogers, personal communication, September 1964.
8. Amidon & Hough, *Interaction Analysis,* p. 137.
9. Carl R. Rogers, *Carl Rogers on Personal Power* (New York: Delacorte, 1977), pp. 91–92.
10. Douglas McGregor, *The Human Side of Enterprise* (New York: McGraw-Hill, 1960).
11. Chris Argyris, *Management and Organizational Development* (New York: McGraw-Hill, 1971); idem, *On Organizations of the Future,* (Beverly Hills: Sage, 1973).
12. Warren G. Bennis, *Organizational Development: Its Nature, Origin and Prospects* (Reading, MA: Addison-Wesley, 1967).
13. R. Likert, *New Patterns of Management* (New York: McGraw-Hill, 1961); idem, *The Human Organization* (New York: McGraw-Hill, 1967).

Unit Exercises
Multiple-Choice Items

Answers are on page 192.

1. General areas of agreement that should be established between teacher and supervisor are:

    a. teacher's goals for the year.
    b. mutual concerns.
    c. common rationale.
    d. teaching strategies to be considered.
    e. All the above are correct.

2. From the following, choose the *best* remark for getting the conference down to business:

    a. How do you feel?
    b. How's your family?
    c. You had a good lesson.
    d. Let's take a look at the data I recorded.
    e. You need to be stricter.

3. Which of the following assumptions about teachers are *not* compatible with the authors' view? Most teachers have:

    a. reasonable goals.
    b. access to alternative strategies.
    c. little need for improvement.
    d. preference for democratic supervision.
    e. adequate information and perspective on their own.

4. Major steps in the feedback process are:

    a. provide data.
    b. analyze data.
    c. interpret what is happening.
    d. make decisions on future actions.
    e. All the above are correct.

5. When a teacher asks a supervisor, "What would *you* do?" the supervisor should:

   a. refuse to answer.
   b. describe exactly what to do.
   c. give several alternatives.
   d. encourage the teacher to think of several alternatives.
   e. say, "What would *you* do?"

6. Which of the following fit Carl Rogers's notions of influence and impact (as opposed to power and control)?

   a. Having teachers make their own tape recordings of lessons.
   b. Having teachers turn in lesson plans.
   c. Filing evaluations that are not seen by the teacher.
   d. Giving merit pay.
   e. Asking teachers for feedback about supervisory conferences.

7. A behavior that is either direct or indirect is:

   a. lecturing.
   b. giving directions.
   c. giving praise.
   d. asking questions.
   e. criticizing.

8. Two behaviors from Spaulding's list that would describe the authors' ideal conference are:

   a. respond to internal stimuli.
   b. control.
   c. transact.
   d. seek help.
   e. share.

Problems

The following problems do not have single correct answers. Answers are on pages 193–94. Your answers may differ from these yet be as good or better.

1. Think of a teacher you have known who had a definite problem with classroom management (student discipline). Then (a) list several alternatives this teacher might try. Next (b) write a sen-

tence that you would use in suggesting these alternatives to the teacher.

2. Identify a teaching strategy that is not in the list on page 66—for example, a field trip or committee meetings—and devise a "self-observation" plan a teacher could use to collect data about the lesson.

3. Consider the categories suggested by Spaulding (p. 70). Put them in the first column of a three-column list. In the second column, suggest (with a brief phrase) a common student behavior in the classroom that fits each category. In the third column, identify teacher behaviors in conferences with supervisors that would fit each category. For example:

Spaulding's list	Student behavior (classroom)	Teacher behavior (conference)
• • •	•	•
Respond to external stimuli	Distracted by another student sharpening pencil	Interrupting conference to deal with a student in the hall
• •	•	•

Unit III

Techniques of Classroom Observation

Overview

In order to have persuasive data available in feedback conferences, the supervisor needs a range of observation techniques and recording devices. A number of instruments and procedures are described in this unit. Most of them are easily understood and can be used effectively after a little practice. The information they provide for the teacher and the supervisor is a central element of the clinical cycle.

Objectives

The purpose of this unit is to help you develop:

A repertoire of data-recording techniques.
Means for selecting an appropriate observation system for a given concern.
Understanding of the strengths and limitations of the various systems.
Recognition of the need for regular, systematic observation and a variety of sources of data.

6

The Technique of Selective Verbatim

"Except in special instances in which some quality of timing or of sound or of sight evolved as a salient supervisory issue, written data have proven most useful and most wieldy to clinical supervisors. Perhaps the greatest advantage of a written record . . . is that Teacher and Supervisor can assimilate it most rapidly and most easily; the eye can incorporate, almost instantaneously, evidence that took a relatively long time to unfold in the lesson."—Robert Goldhammer

What teachers and students say to one another has a major effect on the learning process. Therefore, an important skill in teacher supervision is the ability to listen and record what is being said during classroom visitation.

Selective verbatim is one technique for recording events in the classroom. As the term implies, the supervisor makes a written record of exactly what is said, that is, a verbatim transcript. Not all verbal events are recorded, however. Supervisor and teacher select beforehand certain kinds of verbal events to be written down; in this sense, the verbatim record is intended to be "selective." Most of our discussion of the selective verbatim technique is concerned with identifying verbal interactions that reflect effective or ineffective teaching and thus are worth recording as part of clinical supervision.

Selective verbatim usually is done by the supervisor while the teacher's class is in progress. This is not a necessary requirement. If an audio or video recording of a class session is available (see chapter 8), a selective verbatim can be made from the recording.

As we use the term, selective verbatim implies a word-for-word transcription of particular verbal statements. Suppose a supervisor is recording a teacher's questions, and the teacher asks, "What do we call animals that live exclusively off plants; you know, we have a certain name for these animals, does anyone know it?" If the supervisor writes, "What is the name of animals that live exclusively off plants?" this is not a verbatim transcription.

Selective verbatim has a number of obvious benefits and advantages as a technique of classroom observation. We mention four of them here. First, providing a teacher with a selective verbatim transcript focuses the teacher's attention on what he or she says to students or on what students say to the teacher. As a result, the teacher is sensitized to the *verbal* process in teaching. All other classroom events are screened out by the transcript.

The second advantage of selective verbatim is that it *is* selective. Teacher and supervisor do not need to respond to all aspects of the teaching-learning process, just a few simple verbal behaviors. Teachers who are trying to improve their instruction are more successful if they do not try to change many aspects of behavior at once. Changing a few behaviors at a time encourages further changes. For example, we have experienced the sense of accomplishment teachers get when they realize they are using an annoying verbal mannerism, such as "you know" or "uh," and achieve control over it. This sense of control and change motivates further, more substantial changes in teaching behavior.

A third advantage of selective verbatim is that it provides an objective, noninterpretive record of the teacher's behavior. In "live" classroom teaching, the teacher may be so caught up in the process of teaching that he or she may not hear the actual words. Even if the teacher hears, the verbal events occur rapidly and are forgotten before the teacher can reflect on their meaning and effectiveness. In contrast, selective verbatim holds a "verbal" mirror up to the teacher, which can be analyzed at the teacher's convenience.

Finally, selective verbatim has the advantage of being relatively simple to use. All that the supervisor needs is a pencil and pad of paper. Also, the verbatim transcript is made while the supervisor is in the process of observing the teacher's classroom. There is no need to do additional transcription work after the observation period.

To provide a balanced view, we should mention several potential problems that can occur with selective verbatim. A teacher who knows in advance what verbal behaviors will be recorded (e.g., the teacher's questions, verbal mannerisms, praise statements) may become self-conscious in using the behaviors. Just knowing that a supervisor will observe verbal praise, for example, may increase a teacher's use of this behavior. It is to be hoped that the teacher will gradually internalize verbal praise as a technique and use it even when the supervisor is not around.

We find in practice that teachers generally do not become self-conscious when selective verbatim is used. They are not aware of their verbal behavior and *want* to learn more about what they say and what their students say.

Another potential problem with selective verbatim arises from its "selectivity." The larger context of classroom interaction is lost if teacher and supervisor focus too narrowly on verbal behavior. A teacher may look at a selective verbatim of praise statements and dismiss them with, "Oh, I see I used verbal praise ten times. I guess that's pretty good." The analysis needs to go further to explore such questions as whether the praise was given to students who deserved it and whether it was not used when it should have been. In-depth analysis of this kind requires that the supervisor record, at least mentally, the entire flow of the lesson. A skillful supervisor is one who simplifies the teaching process by focusing the teacher's attention on a few aspects of teaching yet relates these aspects to the total context in which the behaviors occurred.

Still another problem with selective verbatim is that teacher or supervisor may select apparently trivial verbal behaviors for observation. Both supervisor and teacher need to explore why each identified verbal behavior is worth recording and analyzing. If a rationale cannot be given, they must consider whether scarce supervisory time should be used in recording the particular verbal behavior.

Occasionally supervisors find that they cannot keep up with the verbal interaction. It simply occurs too fast to record. In this situation we recommend that supervisors use a symbol such as a line to indicate where they stopped recording temporarily. It is better to record a few verbal statements word for word than to paraphrase or shorten what was said.

Teacher Questions (Technique 8)

Asking questions may well be the most important activity in which teachers engage. Aschner, for example, called the teacher a "professional question maker" and claimed that the asking of questions is "one of the basic ways by which the teacher stimulates student thinking and learning." [1]

Certainly teachers rely on question asking as a staple of their teaching repertoire. A half century ago, Stevens found that high school teachers asked almost four hundred questions during an average school day. [2] Unbelievable as this may seem, it is also mentioned in studies of more recent vintage. Floyd found that a sample of primary school teachers asked an average of 348 questions each during a school day. [3] In Moyer's study, elementary school teachers asked an average of 180 questions each in a science lesson. [4] In Schreiber's study, fifth-grade teachers asked an average of 64 questions each in a thirty-minute social studies lesson. [5] At the high school level, Bellack found that "the core of the teaching sequence found in the classrooms studied is a teacher's question, a pupil's response, and, more often than not, a teacher's reaction to that response." [6] These studies suggest that if a teacher and a supervisor can observe only a single aspect of classroom interaction, they might be well advised to focus on the teacher's question-asking behavior.

Technique

The supervisor's task is to make a written record of each question asked by the teacher. Since teachers typically ask many questions, the supervisor might ask the teacher to estimate the length of the lesson. Then the supervisor uses time sampling, which means that the supervisor observes samples of the lesson (e.g., the first three minutes of the lesson, five minutes in the middle of the lesson, and three minutes at the end of the lesson). Obviously, if you are planning to observe the teacher's use of questions, you will want to select a lesson in which this verbal behavior occurs with some frequency.

It seems a simple matter to decide what is or is not a question. "How many kilometers in a mile?" is obviously a question. But how about "Johnny gave a good answer, didn't he?" or "Sue, won't you stop fidgeting in your seat?" or "I'd like somebody to tell me how many kilometers there are in a mile." The latter example is a declarative statement, not an interrogative, yet it clearly has the intent of a question.

To avoid confusion, we suggest a simple rule. If the teacher's statement is asked in a questioning manner or has the intent of a question, include it in the transcript. There is no harm in including

ambiguous examples, but omitting them may cause a teacher to overlook a significant aspect of his or her question-asking behavior.

What follows are two selective verbatims based on observation of
two fifth-grade teachers. The teachers assigned students to read the
same brief handout on the behavior patterns and environment of the
wolf, followed by a question-and-answer session to help the students
review and think about what they had just read.

Teacher 1
  1. Now, what do we know about this animal? What do
     you know about the wolf? You can refer back to
     this little ditto, if you'd like. Jeff?
  2. Next?
  3. Mike?
  4. Heather?
  5. Now Jeff just said that sometimes livestock . . .
     people or farmers hate them because they kill
     their livestock. Would livestock be small
     animals? What do you think?
  6. Terry?
  7. John?
  8. Mike?
  9. Terry, again?
 10. Jeff?
 11. Jerry?
 12. Who said that, Jerry? Was there a quote or
     something in that article?
 13. Do you remember the man's name?
 14. Do you know something? Last night, after we read
     this article, after school, Jeff said, "Gee Mr.
     Edwards, I think I've seen that name, or
     something." He went right down to the library
     and brought back this book, and it's by the same
     man. Jeff, did you have a chance to look at that
     last night?
 15. Jeff, does it just concern itself with the wolf?
 16. Does anyone have anything else to say about what
     we already know?

Teacher 2
  1. What do you know about the Arctic and that kind
     of area that would lead you to believe that a
     dog would have to be more strong there than he
     would have to be, say, here? Dana?
  2. Pam?

```
 3. What kind of work does he have to do?
 4. Terry?
 5. Karen?
 6. Why do the dogs work harder in the north than
    they work here? John?
 7. Why don't our dogs have to work?
 8. What don't we need done here?
 9. Allen?
10. Doug?
11. Why do you suppose the Eskimos don't have
    machines? Joey?
12. Do you think so? Does anyone have another idea
    about why they don't, 'cause there's probably
    more than one idea?
13. Why would they be primitive? Pam?
14. Wanda?
15. It mentioned in the stories that wolves traveled
    in packs, in groups. Why do you suppose they do?
    What do you suppose is their reason for doing
    this? Joe?
```

Exhibit 6.1. Selective verbatims of fifth-grade teachers' questions

Data Analysis

When teachers examine selective verbatims of their questions, they often observe the following behaviors:

Cognitive level of question. Teachers' questions can be classified into two categories: "fact" and "higher cognitive." Fact questions require students to recall facts or information stated in the curriculum materials. Higher cognitive questions (sometimes called "thought" questions), in contrast, require students to *think* about what they have read and state their own ideas.

Fact questions and higher cognitive questions are not always easy to distinguish from one another. For example, a student may be asked to recall a fact stated in the assigned reading. The student may not be able to recall the fact but deduces it, using higher cognitive processes and other information he knows. A question that is higher cognitive in form (e.g., a "why?" question) may actually be a "fact" question if the student simply repeats an idea he heard or read elsewhere.

It is apparent that the first teacher in exhibit 6.1 is emphasizing fact questions as indicated by phrases like "What do we know?" "Who said that?" and "Did you . . . look at that last night?" In contrast, the second teacher focuses on higher cognitive processes, as indicated by phrases like "What would lead you to believe?" "Why?" and "Does anyone have another idea?"

There is no convincing research evidence that one kind of question is superior to the other.[7] Their effectiveness is probably best judged by examining the teacher's intent for the lesson in which the questions occurred. If the teacher's intent is to stimulate students to think about what they have read, it seems reasonable to expect that the teacher will emphasize higher cognitive questions and use fact questions only when the student's information base is weak.

Amount of information. Fact questions can be classified further into "narrow" and "broad," depending on the amount of information called for in the question. For example, the first teacher in exhibit 6.1 asked, "What do you know about the wolf?" This is an example of a *broad* fact question. "Do you remember the man's name?" is an example of a *narrow* fact question because it asks for only one bit of information. Teachers sometimes ask a series of narrow fact questions—a practice that uses up much class time and is teacher-centered—when one broad question might be sufficient.

Redirection. Teachers can call on one student to answer each question, or they can ask several students to respond to a particular question. That is, they can "redirect" the question. Both teachers in exhibit 6.1 used this technique, usually by simply naming the student they wished to respond. Higher cognitive questions are redirected more easily than fact questions because the former usually do not have a single correct answer. Redirection is a useful technique for increasing student participation and eliciting a variety of ideas for students to consider.

Probing questions. These are "follow-up" questions designed to improve a student's initial response to a teacher question. They are not easy to detect in a selective verbatim, unless the supervisor makes special note of them (perhaps by placing a P beside each such question). The following is a complete verbatim of the events that transpired when the second teacher in exhibit 6.1 asked questions 6 and 7.

> *Teacher*:   Why do the dogs work harder in the north than they work here? John?
>
> *John*:   Well, most of the dogs here don't really have to work hard, but up north, you know, they have to do all the chores and pull sleds and everything like that.

[P] *Teacher*:   Why don't our dogs have to work?

John: They're house pets, and we do most of the work ourselves, and we don't need stuff done like they do up there.

[P] *Teacher*:   What don't we need done here?

John: We don't need dogs to pull things here. We have cars, but the Eskimos don't, so they use dogs.

The teacher's two probing questions helped John give a more complete and specific answer to the initial question.

Teachers often are unaware that they accept or overlook poor responses to their questions. A record of their probing questions provides one indication of whether this is a problem. Absence of probing questions suggests lack of attention to student responses, whereas liberal use of this technique suggests that the teacher is listening carefully to what students say and is challenging them to do their best work.

Multiple questions. The practice of asking several questions in a row can be spotted easily in a selective verbatim. Note that the first teacher begins his lesson by asking two questions in succession: "Now, what do we know about this animal? What do you know about the wolf?" The same teacher also asks multiple questions in the fifth and twelfth recorded statements. The second teacher asks multiple questions in the twelfth and fifteenth recorded statements.

Teachers usually engage in this behavior when they are "thinking on their feet." They may try various phrasings and ideas before they hit upon a question to which they wish students to respond. A teacher who asks multiple questions habitually should examine this practice to determine whether it is distracting or confusing to students. The teacher can avoid asking multiple questions by preparing questions in advance of the actual lesson.

Teacher Feedback (Technique 9)

Research, as well as everyday observation, demonstrates that feedback has an effect on the learning process. If we are learning a new skill, we need feedback to know how correctly or well we are performing the skill. Without feedback, we may simply practice bad habits or terminate training too soon. Praise or negative remarks as a particular form of feedback also may affect our behavior, especially our motivation to learn.

Jonn Zahorik, in his study of classroom feedback behavior of teachers, found that teachers' verbal feedback tends to be constricted.[8] Only a few kinds of feedback are used regularly. Zahorik found that the most frequent form of feedback to students was simply to repeat the student's answer to a question. Ned Flanders also found that teachers' most common form of feedback consists of simple repetition of what the pupil has said.[9] Flanders and educators in general have advocated that teachers learn how to extend the amount and variety of feedback they provide to students.

Praise and criticism as feedback are of particular interest to educational researchers. In their review of research on criticism, Rosenshine and Furst found evidence to support the generalization that "teachers who use extreme amounts or forms of criticism usually have classes which achieve less in most subject areas."[10] They also found, however, that mild forms of criticism did not produce similar results. They note that "there is no evidence to support a claim that teachers should avoid telling a student he was wrong or should avoid giving academic directions."[11]

In the same review, Rosenshine and Furst did not find a relationship between student achievement and variations in teachers' use of praise statements. Research studies not included in their review, however, especially research on behavior modification, demonstrate that teacher use of praise statements ("positive reinforcers" is the technical term) has a positive effect on student performance. The findings from this line of research also suggest that it is not helpful, in many instances, to provide negative feedback (e.g., criticism, rebukes) when students engage in socially undesirable behavior. The rule of thumb seems to be: Provide positive feedback when the student exhibits desirable behavior; avoid negative feedback when the students engage in undesirable behavior.

Technique

As supervisor, you need to arrange with the teacher to observe a sample of classroom instruction in which there is ample opportunity for verbal interchange between teacher and students. During the classroom instruction, you record the teacher's verbal feedback statements. It also may be useful to record the immediately preceding student remark or action that prompted the feedback. Another option is to make note of the affective context: Was the verbal feedback hostile in tone? enthusiastic? automatic?

As with question classification, it is not always an easy matter to decide whether a particular teacher remark is an instance of verbal feedback. You will need to rely on your judgment to determine whether a particular remark is likely to be *perceived* by a student as feedback on his or her behavior. Thus, the supervisor needs to be a close observer of students' reactions and the total instructional context when making the selective verbatim.

Exhibit 6.2 presents a selective verbatim of a junior high school teacher's feedback statements. The lesson was organized around an article about population explosion that the students had been asked to read.

T: All right. Could someone tell me what the report was about? Ann?

S: Well, it was about birth control.

T: Birth control?

S: Uh, population explosion.

. . .

S: It was about the population explosion, but it was also about limits. It made a lot of predictions, like we won't have room to get around, and there's not going to be any room to plant crops.

T: <u>I'm glad you remembered that the author said that these were "predictions."</u> Why do you think I'm <u>glad you remembered that</u> the author used the word "predictions?"

. . .

S: I also heard that they're going to have a farm under the sea, for sea-farming.

T: <u>Who's "they"?</u>

S: Well . . . the scientists.

. . .

S: And as the years go by, cars will get better and better.

T: <u>Are you sure?</u>

S: Well, I'm not certain, but pretty sure.

T: <u>Pretty sure. This is kind of what I wanted you to</u> <u>get out of this article. These are your opinions,</u>

your predictions of what might happen. And they
sound pretty good to me, and I'll bank on them to
a certain extent, but something might happen to
the automobile industry so that your predictions
wouldn't come true.
                              . . .

T: Who made that statement that was quoted in the
   article?

S: Professor Kenneth E. F. Watt.

T: Professor Kenneth E. F. Watt is saying it. Do we
   know that what he's saying is worthwhile?

S: Well, Professor Kenneth E. F. Watt isn't the only
   one that is making these predictions. There's
   probably thousands of people making these
   predictions.

T: Yes, that's a good point, Rodney. We can have
   some faith in what he's predicting because others
   are making similar predictions.
                              . . .

T: Why, throughout the whole world, are there so
   many people having so many children? Did you ever
   stop to think about it? Steve?

S: When the children grow up, they want children.
   Then when those children grow up, then they get
   more children, and that goes on and on.

T: Steve, I'm not sure I'm following you. Could you
   clarify your idea a bit? Why do people want to
   have so many children?
                              . . .

T: I thought the ideas you had to contribute were a
   lot more interesting than the article itself.

Exhibit 6.2. Selective verbatim of teacher feedback

Data Analysis

The teacher and the supervisor can examine a selective verbatim of
feedback behavior from several perspectives, including the following:
  Amount. The simplest analysis you can make of the selective verbatim is to determine the frequency with which the teacher provides
feedback. You may observe teachers who provide little or no feedback

to their students. These teachers tend to use a very directive style of instruction; their primary concern is to impart knowledge (perhaps with too little concern about whether students are "receiving" the knowledge). Other teachers make extensive use of feedback. They tend to be more responsive to students and to encourage teacher-student interaction.

Variety. Of concern here is whether the teacher relies on a few limited forms of feedback (research indicates that this is what most teachers do) or whether they provide a variety of feedback. As noted, Flanders found that teachers most often provide feedback on students' ideas by acknowledging them.[12] Acknowledgment takes the form of repeating the student's idea virtually verbatim. Flanders has shown that student ideas can be acknowledged and used more effectively, for example, by doing the following:

a. *modifying* the idea by rephrasing or conceptualizing it in the teacher's own words
b. *applying* the idea by using it to reach an inference or take the next step in a logical analysis of a problem
c. *comparing* the idea with other ideas expressed earlier by the students or the teacher
d. *summarizing* what was said by an individual student or group of students

Teacher verbal feedback also can be analyzed to determine whether there is variety in the teacher's use of praise and critical or corrective remarks.

Another perspective for analyzing variety of teacher feedback is to determine the nature of the student responses that elicited the feedback statement. Does the teacher limit feedback to the information contained in the student's answer? Or does the teacher extend feedback to include the student's ideas, behavior, and feelings? Research conducted by Flanders and others indicates that teachers seldom acknowledge students' feelings, although most educators would agree that feelings—and other aspects of the affective domain—are an important part of the instructional process.

Specificity. Teachers tend to give simple forms of feedback, saying, "Good," "Yes, that's right," "No," or "Fine." Flanders, Zahorik, and other educators suggest that teachers should develop the habit of elaborating on their feedback by giving students an explanation for their praise or criticism. "Good, you lined up your columns of numbers very well that time" is much more specific and more helpful to a student than just saying "Good." Similarly, "I'm not sure you answered my question; listen carefully while I ask the question again" is probably more helpful than a noncommittal "Uh-huh" or "No, does anyone else have an idea?" Even a quick inspection of a selective verbatim should help a teacher see the extent to which he or she uses simple versus elaborated forms of feedback.

Teacher Directions and Structuring Statements (Technique 10)

An important part of the teacher's role is to *manage* students' learning. Management involves giving directions and structuring the learning situation—that is, telling students what to study, how to complete an assignment or carry out an activity, what is important to remember, what to do in preparation for a test.

The findings of research support the common-sense notion that the manner in which teachers give directions to students or whether teachers give directions at all has an effect on student achievement. Rosenshine and Furst reviewed research on teachers' use of structuring statements, which can take such forms as (1) statements that provide an overview for what is to happen in a lesson; (2) summaries of what has happened in a lesson; (3) statements that indicate to a class when the teacher is switching from one topic to the next; and (4) verbal cues that emphasize the importance of some point in the lesson (e.g., "Pay particular attention to what happens next in the experiment"). Research studies consistently have found higher levels of student achievement associated with teachers who make use of structuring statements.[13]

Similar research has not been done on the effects of teacher directions, but it seems obvious that teachers who give vague, ambiguous directions will confuse students and interfere with their learning. Indirect evidence that this is true comes from research on teachers' overall clarity. Seven studies of clarity reviewed by Rosenshine and Furst found a positive relationship between the clarity of a teacher's presentation and measures of student learning.[14]

Technique

It is probably best to observe a teacher's directions and structuring statements in the context of a complete lesson. Therefore, as supervisor, you need to speak beforehand with the teacher to determine when to begin observing and approximately how long the lesson will last. Then, during the lesson, you make a selective verbatim of each set of directions and structuring statements made by the teacher. Most of these statements usually occur at the beginning and the end of the lesson, so you need to be especially observant at these times.

Exhibit 6.3 presents a composite of lessons in which teachers gave directions and structuring comments. We used this approach, rather than presenting the selective verbatim of one teacher, to show the variety of forms that directions and structuring comments can take.

1. Make sure you write this down in your notebook.
2. OK. Most of you have finished. We will go on to the next poem.
3. Would someone please read the introduction?
4. Class, let's have an orderly discussion today. When you want to talk, please raise your hand and I'll call on you.
5. The report we're going to read today is about apartheid in South Africa.
6. The film we just saw on how glass is made illustrates very well some of the points that were covered in the book we're using in this course.
7. Yes, electric cars are one of the really important ways we might be able to control air pollution in the future. You might want to remember that when you write your science-fiction stories.
8. OK. Today I've shown you three different ways you can do calculations. First, we have the slide rule. Second, you can use the desk calculator. And third—does anyone remember what the third method is?
9. Let's act out this scene from the book. Who wants to be Huck Finn? Who wants to be Jim? . . . Now that we have all the characters, I want the rest of you to watch closely. See how well they do the scene as Mark Twain wrote it.
10. Now that you've finished role playing, let's talk about it. How do you feel now about Huck Finn?

Exhibit 6.3 Examples of teacher directions and structuring statements

Data Analysis

As with teacher feedback, teacher and supervisor can observe *amount, variety,* and *specificity* of directions and structuring comments. In addition, it is helpful to observe whether the statements are clear, that is whether they tell the student precisely what to do.

As we stated, teacher directions and structuring comments can take a variety of forms, for example:

1. An overview of the lesson about to be presented to the class
2. The objectives and purpose of the lesson
3. Cueing remarks that focus the student's attention on key points in the lesson
4. A summary of what was covered in the lesson
5. Statements that relate the lesson to curriculum content previously covered or to events outside the classroom
6. Directions concerning what students are to do while the lesson is in progress, after the lesson is completed, or if a student completes an assignment while other students are still working
7. Reinforcement of key directions and structuring comments by repeating them in another format (e.g., through a handout, on the blackboard, or by an overhead projector)

This list is not exhaustive, but it does illustrate the range of teacher comments and actions you can include in a selective verbatim of directions and structuring comments.

Notes

1. M. J. Aschner, "Asking Questions to Trigger Thinking," *NEA Journal* 50 (1961): 44–46.
2. R. Stevens, "The Question as a Measure of Efficiency in Instruction: A Critical Study of Classroom Practice," *Teachers College Contributions to Education*, no. 48 (1912).
3. W. D. Floyd, "An Analysis of the Oral Questioning Activity in Selected Colorado Primary Classrooms" (Ph.D. diss., Colorado State College, 1960).
4. J. R. Moyer, "An Exploratory Study of Questioning in the Instructional Processes in Selected Elementary Schools" (Ph.D. diss., Columbia University, 1966).
5. J. E. Schreiber, "Teachers' Question-Asking Techniques in Social Studies" (Ph.D. diss., University of Iowa, 1967).
7. Barak Rosenshine and Norma Furst, "Research on Teacher Performance Criteria," in *Research in Teacher Education: A Symposium*, ed. B. O. Smith (Englewood Cliffs, NJ: Prentice-Hall, 1971), 37–72.

8. John A. Zahorik, "Classroom Feedback Behavior of Teachers," *Journal of Educational Research*, 62 (1968): 147–50.

9. Ned A. Flanders, *Analyzing Teaching Behavior* (Reading, MA: Addison-Wesley, 1970).

10. Rosenshine and Furst, "Teacher Performance Criteria," p. 51.

11. Ibid.

12. Flanders, *Analyzing Teaching Behavior*.

13. Rosenshine and Furst, "Teacher Performance Criteria," pp. 51–52.

14. Ibid., pp. 44–45.

7

Observational Records Based on Seating Charts

"These seating chart techniques look simple, but they're not. True, all the supervisor gives you to look at is a seating chart with lines and arrows all over it. But they tell you a lot about what happened in your lesson. You can see that your teaching is following a definite pattern. Then the question you need to ask yourself is, Is this a good or a bad pattern, something I want to change or something I want to keep on doing?"—Comment of a high school teacher

Several techniques for observing teacher and student behavior make use of seating charts. This family of observation instruments is sometimes called Seating Chart Observation Records (SCORE).

One of the main advantages of SCORE instruments is that they are based on classroom seating charts. Since teachers use seating charts in their daily work, they usually find it easy to interpret SCORE data.

SCORE instruments have several other advantages. They enable the supervisor to condense a large amount of information about classroom behavior on a single sheet of paper. SCORE instruments can be created on the spot to suit the individual teacher's concerns. They are easy to use and interpret. Moreover, they get at important aspects of classroom behavior, such as students' level of attentiveness and how teachers distribute their time among students in the class. A special benefit of SCORE instruments is that they enable teacher and supervisor to spotlight individual students in the class, at the same time observing what the class as a whole is doing.

SCORE instruments do have several limitations and disadvantages. They simplify the teaching process by isolating certain behaviors for observation; but unless these behaviors are related to the total teaching-learning context, the teacher may draw simplistic conclusions from the data. Another hazard is that teacher or supervisor may select trivial behaviors for observation. As a supervisor, you should also be aware that sometimes classroom behavior will "speed up" or become chaotic. In this situation, you may need to modify or temporarily abandon the data-collection process.

At Task (Technique 11)

The at-task technique was developed in the 1960s by Frank McGraw at Stanford University.[1] McGraw devised a system of classroom observation that used a 35-mm camera, remotely controlled. From the front corner of the room the camera took a picture of the total class every ninety seconds, using a wide-angle lens. The photos were developed and enlarged. The observer was then provided with a set of pictures of a classroom during a given time period (e.g., twenty pictures to represent a thirty-minute lesson).

A variety of results were obtained. Some looked like the films formerly shown in nickelodeons, where the students gradually move from a position of sitting erect at their desks to a position of sleeping with their heads on their desks, back to a position of sitting and looking attentive. Other collections of pictures showed students working feverishly on matters that had nothing to do with the task at hand, or vacant from their seats talking to their neighbors, or engaged in a variety of actions the teacher regarded as inappropriate.

The data obtained from the pictures were valuable for the teacher in understanding individual students. But the method of collecting data was so demanding, expensive, and time-consuming that experiments were conducted using alternative methods. Ultimately a paper-and-pencil technique was developed to provide much the same data as the 35-mm camera. This paper-and-pencil technique has come to be known as "at task." A completed "at task" is shown on page 110.

Research studies have demonstrated that student at-task behavior is an important factor in learning. This finding has intuitive appeal. It seems obvious that the more a student attends to the tasks presented by the teacher, the more he or she will learn. The correlation between at-task behavior and learning is not perfect, however. One student may attend carefully to a teacher's lecture or to the words in a textbook, yet end up confused and unable to master the lesson content. Another student may work eagerly on the assigned task but may fail to learn because he or she is using incorrect or inappropriate behaviors; for example, using "regrouping" incorrectly in computation problems. Nonetheless, if students are at-task, one can conclude with some confidence that learning is taking place.

Because there is a clear link between student at-task behavior and learning, the at-task observational technique is probably the most important of the SCORE procedures.

Technique

The intent of at-task observation is to provide data on whether individual students during a classroom activity were engaged in the task or tasks that the teacher indicated were appropriate. Before an observer can use this technique, then, he must be acquainted with what the teacher expects the students to be doing during a given classroom period. In other words, the teacher rather than the supervisor defines what constitutes at-task behavior.

Typical at-task behaviors are reading, listening, answering questions, drawing a map, working cooperatively to complete a group project. Those classrooms where one task is expected of all students usually present no problem, but where students are able to do a variety of tasks some preparation is necessary before the supervisor can use this technique. If the variety of tasks is too complex, teacher and supervisor may choose to limit the observation to one group or section of the classroom.

To use the at-task technique the supervisor must complete these seven steps:

1. Stations himself in a section of the room where he is able to observe all students.
2. Constructs a chart that resembles a seating pattern of the students in the room that day.
3. Indicates on the chart the sex and some other identifying characteristic of each student. The latter is necessary when the students are not known to the supervisor.
4. Creates a legend to represent at-task behavior and each type of inappropriate behavior observed. A typical legend might be

      A: At task

      B: Stalling

      C: Other schoolwork than that requested by the teacher

      D: Out of seat

      E: Talking to neighbors

5.   Systematically examines the behavior of each student for a few seconds in order to determine whether the student is at task, that is, doing what the teacher considers appropriate. If so, indicates this by marking a 1*A* in the box on the seating chart meant to represent the student. Figure 1 indicates that this is the first observation; the letter *A* refers to at-task behavior. If the student is not at task, the observer indicates this by recording 1*B*, 1*C*, 1*D*, or 1*E* (using the legend created in step 4).

6.   Repeats step 5 at three- or four-minute intervals for the duration of the lesson using the same letter legend to indicate observed behavior but changing the number to indicate the sequence of observations. For example, 3*A* in a box indicates that the student was at task during the supervisor's third observation.

7.   Indicates time of each set of observations. This is marked somewhere on the chart (e.g., see upper right-hand corner on page 110).

You are advised to follow a few precautions in using the at-task technique. First, avoid forming too many categories for observation. Step 4 (above) listed five categories—at task, stalling, other school-work than that requested by the teacher, out of seat, and talking to neighbors—probably as many categories as you would want to form. Adding more categories complicates observation greatly, and it becomes increasingly difficult for the teacher to interpret the resulting data. In many classroom observations two categories are sufficient: at task and off task.

In using the at-task technique, supervisors sometimes become overly concerned about the accuracy of their observations. It helps to realize that observation of at-task behavior requires a moderate degree of inference. The expression on a child's face may be interpreted as thoughtful reflection about what the teacher is saying or as daydreaming. We suggest you think "probabilistically." If you think it is more probable that the child is engaged in thoughtful reflection than in daydreaming, use the at-task category. If you think it is more probable that the child is daydreaming, indicate this by using one of your off-task codes. You may wish to tell the teacher that the completed chart is, to an extent, subjective. Thus the teacher should look for general patterns rather than question the accuracy of a few isolated observations.

The at-task chart in exhibit 7.1 has one box for each student in the class. The students are identified by name on the chart. If the feedback conference occurs fairly soon after the observation, the teacher should have no difficulty matching students with the boxes even without names. However, if the feedback conference is delayed, you should consider putting students' names in the appropriate boxes of the seating chart. This creates a problem if the teacher does not have a prepared seating chart to assist you and if you don't know the students' names. A simple solution is for the teacher to have students say their names aloud at the beginning of the class period while you jot them down; the student's first or last name should be sufficient.

You may wish to use several different colored pencils or pens to record at-task data. The seating chart can be one color, and the at-task observations can be a different color. This procedure results in a visually pleasing product for the teacher to study and interpret.

Example

An elementary school principal observed a first-grade teacher's reading class. The decision to do an at-task seating chart grew out of a planning conference between the teacher and the principal. Part of this conference is reproduced below:

T: Would you come in and do an At Task in my classroom? Randall and Ronald do nothing but play and talk. I would like to see just how much they really work.

P: Are Randall and Ronald the only ones you want me to observe?

T: No. I have a real immature group this year. You might as well observe all of them.

P: What do you mean by "immature"?

T: Oh, they have very short attention spans, haven't learned to settle down, and they are all talking without permission. In other words, this first grade doesn't really know how to settle down and do some work.

P: Do they seem to understand what you have planned for them?

T: Yes, but they have a hard time settling down to work. Ronald moans and groans most of the time or plays.

P: What kinds of behavior should I observe for the At Task? What categories should I use?

T: Before I forget, remember some of my children are out of the room for music at the time you're coming.

P: That's right. I'll put it on my checklist so I won't forget it.

T: Check to see if they're out of their seats, talking, playing, or at task. They will also be reading to my aide or to me.

P: I'll make note of the reading aide, and I'll see you tomorrow.

For the purpose of this observation, at-task behavior was defined as independent reading in a workbook at one's seat (*A*) or as reading with the teacher or aide (*B*). The principal also recorded several other categories of behavior: out of seat (*C*); talking (*D*); out of room (*E*); playing (*F*). The categories are shown in the legend in exhibit 7.1, together with the completed at-task seating chart. Exhibit 7.2 presents a data summary of children's at-task behavior.

Data Analysis

Exhibit 7.2 provides a convenient summary of the observations recorded on the seating chart (exhibit 7.1). The teacher can see at a glance how many children were engaged in each category of behavior—either at a particular point in time or summed across all the time samples.

Analysis of at-task data is illustrated nicely by the feedback conference that occurred between the principal and the first-grade teacher. Part of this conference is reproduced below:

T: Let's see. Randall was at task once. Ronald was, too. Here is a shocker! Liz, Laura, and Sharon do a lot of visiting. I can see where I need to do some changes in the seating.

P: That may solve some of your talking and visiting problems.

T: Boy, from nine-twenty to nine-thirty-six five of my students are out to music. This only leaves seven to work with. Gee, I only worked with two children, and the aide worked with one.

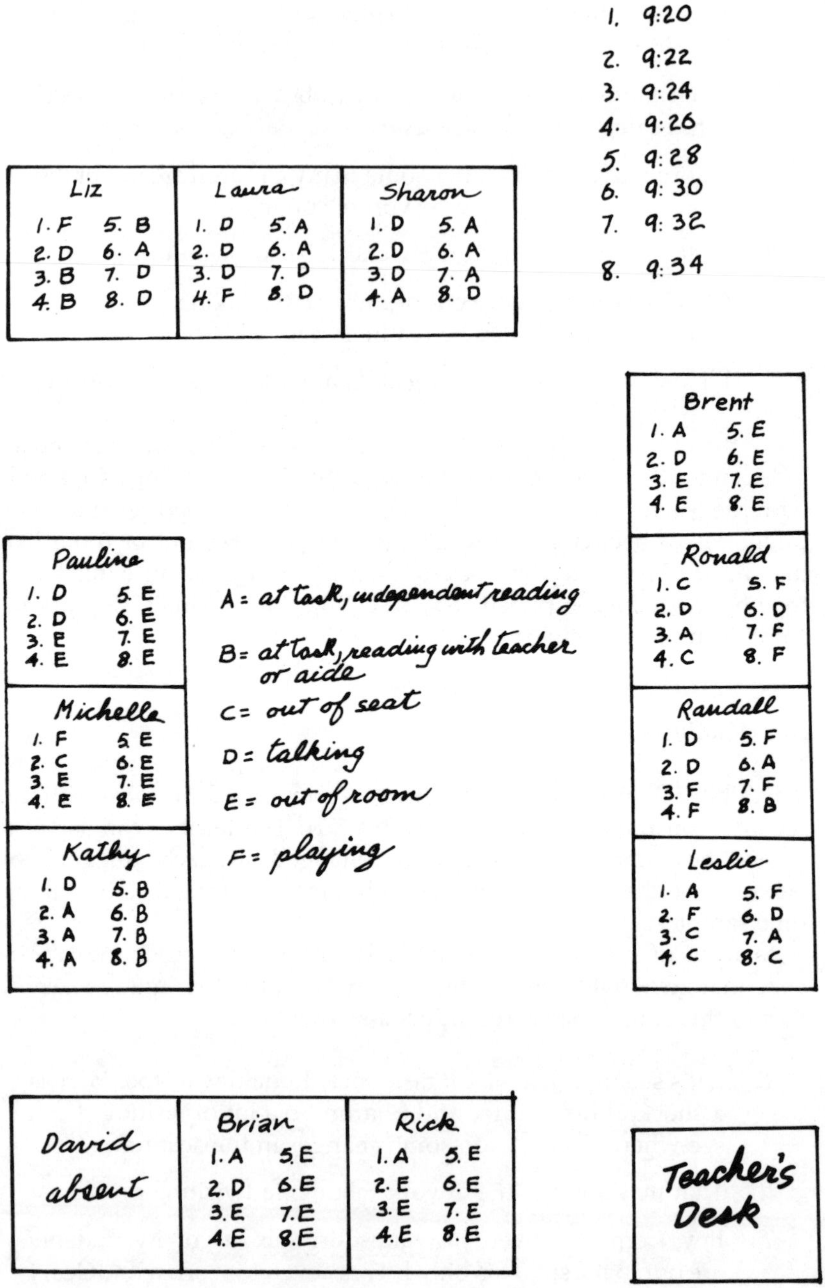

	1.	9:20
	2.	9:22
	3.	9:24
	4.	9:26
	5.	9:28
	6.	9:30
	7.	9:32
	8.	9:34

Liz
1. F	5. B
2. D	6. A
3. B	7. D
4. B	8. D

Laura
1. D	5. A
2. D	6. A
3. D	7. D
4. F	8. D

Sharon
1. D	5. A
2. D	6. A
3. D	7. A
4. A	8. D

Brent
1. A	5. E
2. D	6. E
3. E	7. E
4. E	8. E

Ronald
1. C	5. F
2. D	6. D
3. A	7. F
4. C	8. F

Pauline
1. D	5. E
2. D	6. E
3. E	7. E
4. E	8. E

Michelle
1. F	5. E
2. C	6. E
3. E	7. E
4. E	8. E

Kathy
1. D	5. B
2. A	6. B
3. A	7. B
4. A	8. B

Randall
1. D	5. F
2. D	6. A
3. F	7. F
4. F	8. B

Leslie
1. A	5. F
2. F	6. D
3. C	7. A
4. C	8. C

A = at task, independent reading

B = at task, reading with teacher or aide

C = out of seat

D = talking

E = out of room

F = playing

David absent

Brian
1. A	5. E
2. D	6. E
3. E	7. E
4. E	8. E

Rick
1. A	5. E
2. E	6. E
3. E	7. E
4. E	8. E

Teacher's Desk

Exhibit 7.1. At-task seating chart

BEHAVIOR	9:20	9:22	9:24	9:26	9:28	9:30	9:32	9:34	TOTAL	%
A. At task – independent reading	4	1	2	2	2	4	2	0	17	18%
B. At task – reading with teacher or aide	0	0	1	1	2	1	1	2	8	8%
C. Out of seat	1	1	1	2	0	0	0	1	6	6%
D. Talking	5	8	2	0	0	2	2	3	22	23%
E. Out of room	0	1	5	5	5	5	5	5	31	32%
F. Playing	2	1	1	2	3	0	2	1	12	13%

Exhibit 7.2. Summary of At-task data from Exhibit 7.1

P: It seems as though quite a few of your students are gone at one time.

T: Yes, I should try to work with these students before they go to music.

P: That's a good idea! In that way you can usually have them read to you every day.

T: Maybe I could ask the aide to have Kathy only read a few pages and then listen to someone else.

P: That sounds great!

T: This doesn't solve my problem with Randall and Ronald. Since Brian and Rick go to music, maybe I could put Ronald at Rick's desk. This way I can get a direct view of him. This also would separate the two boys.

P: This sounds like a good step. Maybe you'll want to keep the boys apart permanently in the classroom.

T: I sure hope this works. If not, I'll find something else.

P: I'm sure you will. You seem to have some good ideas already.

T: I could even have the aide work with Ronald and Randall in reading and have her play some phonics games with them. This would help expand their attention span, too.

P: You're really getting some good ideas. It will be interesting to see how they work out. Maybe I could come back and do an At Task again.

T: Yes, I'd like to see if some of my ideas will help the children settle down, especially Ronald and Randall.

This interaction between principal and teacher illustrates the importance of at-task data in clinical supervision. The data focus the teacher's attention directly on the extent to which students are engaged in productive classroom behavior. If students are not at task, the teacher knows that there is a problem that needs correction. As in the example, teacher and supervisor can develop solutions once the problem has been diagnosed.

In inspecting exhibits 7.1 and 7.2, you might note the rapid change in behavior characteristic of young children. Except for those who left the room, the children were likely to change from one category of behavior to another with each observation. For example, Leslie varied back and forth between behavior categories *A, C, D,* and *F* within the fourteen-minute (9:20 to 9:34) period of observation.

Verbal Flow (Technique 12)

Verbal flow is primarily a technique for recording who is talking to whom. It also is useful for recording categories of verbal interaction—for example, teacher question, student answer, teacher praise, student question. Verbal flow is similar to the technique of selective verbatim (see chapter 6) in that both techniques deal with classroom verbal behavior. Selective verbatim is concerned more with the actual content of the verbal communication, whereas verbal flow identifies the initiators and recipients of the verbal communication and the kind of communication in which they are engaged.

A study by Gregg Jackson and Cecilia Cosca highlights the importance of recording verbal flow data.[2] Their study was sponsored by the U.S. Commission on Civil Rights to determine whether teachers in the southwest distributed their verbal behavior differently among Anglo and Chicano students.[3] Observers recorded verbal behaviors in fourth-, eighth-, tenth-, and twelfth-grade classes in fifty-two schools. A modified form of the Flanders Interaction Analysis System (see chapter 9) was used to classify each verbal interaction and whether it was directed to, or initiated by, an Anglo student or a Chicano student.

Jackson and Cosca found that teachers directed significantly more of their verbal behaviors toward Anglo students than toward Chicano pupils. The most striking results were that "teacher praised or encouraged Anglos 35% more than they did Chicanos, accepted or used Anglo's ideas 40% more than they did those of Chicanos, and directed 21% more questions to Anglos than to Chicanos."[4] The researchers also found that Anglo students initiated more verbal behaviors than did Chicano students. It may be argued that the differences in teacher verbal behaviors reflect the fact that Anglo students in these classrooms were generally higher academic achievers than the Chicano students. Even if true, this means that teachers probably should be directing *more,* not fewer, verbal behaviors to Chicano students.

Research has identified other forms of bias in teacher verbal behaviors. Dunkin and Biddle reached the following conclusions in their review of one of these research studies:

> . . . the majority of both *emitters* and *targets* [of verbal behavior]—whether they be teachers or pupils—are located front and center in the classroom. Thus, pupils who are located around the periphery of the classroom are more likely to be spectators than actors in the classroom drama. It could be, then, that if the teacher wants to encourage participation on the part of a quiet pupil or silence on the part of someone who is noisy, she need merely move the pupil to another location in the room! [5]

Although teachers tend to talk more to students seated closest to them, other "location" biases can occur. For example, one teacher found that he had a tendency to acknowledge more questions from students seated to his right than from students seated to his left. After learning of this tendency, the teacher realized that, in talking to a class, he usually looked to the right side of the classroom. Thus, students seated to this side were in the teacher's central line of vision, whereas students to the left were in his peripheral vision. It occurred to the teacher how frustrated students to his left might be if they had questions but could not ask them because they were out of his line of sight. With this new awareness, the teacher made a conscious effort to distribute eye contact equally to all parts of the classroom. This led to a more equal distribution of verbal behaviors.

Research on discussion groups has identified a number of factors related to differences between students in verbal behavior. In a review of this research Meredith and Joyce Gall found that black students tend to participate less in discussions than white students, and younger students tend to participate less than older students. [6] Also, males tend to initiate more verbal acts than do females. This sex difference has been found to occur even among young children.

Verbal flow is a valuable supervisory technique because it helps teachers discover (1) biases in their own verbal behavior and (2) differences between students in verbal participation. Verbal flow is particularly appropriate when the lesson involves discussion, question-and-answer recitation, or other methods that require many verbal interchanges between teacher and students. It is not appropriate for observing instruction low in verbal interaction (e.g., lecture and independent study).

Technique

As with other SCORE observational instruments, the first step in doing a verbal flow is to make a classroom seating chart. Because of the many seating patterns that can occur in classrooms, we suggest that you not have a standard form; rather, create the seating chart on a blank sheet of paper.

A box is used to represent each student. You can put the students' names in the appropriate box, or if you wish to focus on a particular characteristic, you can just indicate the characteristic. For example, the teacher may suggest in the planning conference that you label each student as male or female; characteristically verbal or nonverbal; and high-achieving, average, or low-achieving. Of course, the teacher will need to tell you the labels that apply to each child. The advantage of this kind of chart is that a teacher can more easily determine whether he or she responds differentially to students who vary in these characteristics.

Arrows are used to indicate the flow of verbal interaction. The base of the arrow indicates the person who initiates a verbal interaction, and the head of the arrow indicates the person to whom the comment is directed.

The teacher is an exception to this procedure. Because the teacher usually initiates most of the verbal interactions, it would be awkward to have an arrow leading from the box that designates the teacher to each student to whom a comment is directed. Arrows would be crisscrossing one another as they made their way from the teacher's box to boxes situated at diverse points of the seating chart. This problem is avoided by placing the arrow completely within the student's box. The base of the arrow should come from the general direction of the teacher. This means that the teacher made these statements directed toward this student.

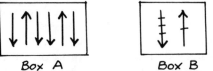

Box A   Box B

One way to keep a verbal flow chart visually simple is to use notches in an arrow to indicate repeated interactions of the same kind. For example, in box A a separate arrow is used to record each interaction. Analysis of these data indicates that the teacher directed four comments to this student, and the student directed two comments back to the teacher. The same data are recorded in box B by two arrows. The arrow indicating the teacher-initiated comment has three notches on it. The arrow indicates one comment, and each notch represents a comment, for a total of four teacher-initiated comments. Similarly, box B indicates a total of two student-initiated comments.

The standard verbal flow chart can be elaborated by using additional categories of observation. The following are possible teacher categories:

   ———➤ +   teacher praise or encouraging remark
   ———➤ −   teacher criticism or negative remark
   ———➤ ?   teacher question
   ——— | teacher asks a question or makes a comment to the class as a whole

Student verbal behaviors also can be differentiated, for example:

   ———➤ √   student volunteered a relevant or correct response
   ———➤ X   student volunteered an irrelevant or incorrect response
   ———➤ ?   student question
   ——— | student comment directed to the class as a whole

The teacher should participate during the planning conference in deciding what categories are to be observed. It is inadvisable to form more than a few categories. Otherwise the recording and interpretation of verbal flow data become unwieldy.

Some supervisors prefer to use an alphabetic notation system rather than arrows. Letters of the alphabet indicate discrete categories of verbal interaction; for example:

Q teacher question
P teacher praise
C teacher criticism
R student volunteered a relevant or correct response
X student volunteered an irrelevant or incorrect response
q student question

Teacher and student behaviors are easily distinguished by the use of upper-case and lower-case letters.

Either arrows or alphabetic notation will get the job done. The choice of one or the other is a matter of preference.

Example

The assistant principal of a high school, one of whose responsibilities is teacher supervision, was asked by a first-year English teacher to determine which students were contributing to classroom and small-group discussions. The teacher's purpose was not to use the supervisor's data to evaluate the students but to learn whether she was influencing students' participation and how nonparticipating students could be encouraged to join the discussion.

Teacher and supervisor agreed that a verbal flow chart was an appropriate technique for collecting the data. The supervisor arranged to visit the teacher's class at a time when a discussion was scheduled.

The verbal flow chart made by the supervisor is presented in exhibit 7.3. Horizontal lines are used to indicate empty desks. Students' sex is indicated by an M or F. The supervisor recorded verbal flow data into four categories: teacher question, student response, teacher positive response, and teacher negative response. Because some students talked among themselves, the supervisor decided to record this behavior by drawing an arrow between the students engaged in such talk. The period of observation was twenty-two minutes.

Data Analysis

Verbal flow data can be analyzed from various perspectives. They include the following:

Seat-location preferences. As we mentioned, some teachers direct more of their attention to students seated in a certain part of the room. This is quite apparent in the teacher's verbal flow chart. As she herself noted, she suffers from tunnel vision. You can see in exhibit 7.3 that she asked most of her questions of students seated directly in her line of sight. Students on either side of her line of sight were ignored. This is a common pattern even among experienced teachers. You also may have noted that comments among students, while the lesson was in progress, occurred only at the periphery of the seating arrangement.

On seeing the verbal flow chart, the teacher commented that she might solve the problem of tunnel vision by seating students closer together, using the available empty seats. Another suggestion is to

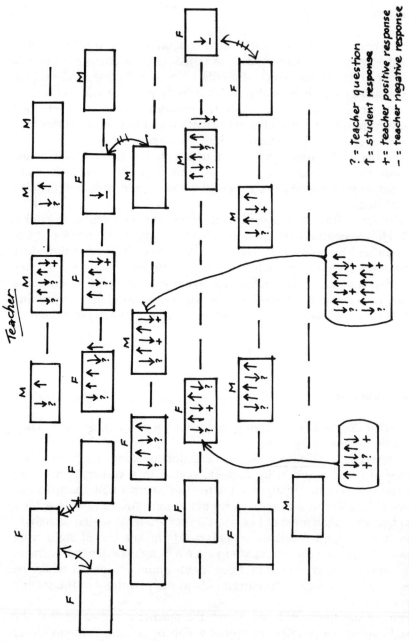

Teacher

? = teacher question
↑ = student response
+ = teacher positive response
– = teacher negative response

Exhibit 7.3. Verbal flow chart

place students in a circular seating arrangement so that everyone can have eye contact with one another.

Student preferences. In exhibit 7.3 students are characterized by sex. One can ask whether the teacher interacted equally with boys and girls, and whether she used each category of verbal behavior equally with them.

The verbal flow chart indicates that thirteen girls and eleven boys were present for the lesson. Of the twenty questions asked by the teacher, twelve (60 percent) were directed to boys, and eight (40 percent) were directed to girls. Of the twelve positive responses by the teacher, eight (66 percent) were directed to boys and four (33 percent) were directed to girls. The two negative responses by the teacher both were directed to girls. Nine of the thirteen girls (70 percent) and four (36 percent) of the eleven boys did not participate in the lessons. These data suggest a sex bias favoring boys.

You might also note in exhibit 7.3 that two students, a boy and a girl, dominated the participation. (The supervisor needed to create additional boxes to contain their data.) Thirty percent of the total number of questions asked by the teacher were directed to these two students. Moreover, they accounted for nearly half the student responses.

Verbal behavior preferences. Verbal flow charts can be inspected to determine how frequently teachers and students use certain behaviors and whether they emphasize certain behaviors more than others. One contrast of interest in exhibit 7.3 is the teacher's use of positive response behavior compared with her use of negative response behavior. Of the teacher's fourteen responses, all but two were positive. The two negative responses were directed toward girls near the periphery of the classroom.

Another possible comparison in exhibit 7.3 is the number of student responses followed by a teacher positive response versus the number of student responses not followed by a teacher positive response. There were thirty-two student responses in the lesson. Of these, twelve (38 percent) were accompanied by a teacher positive response. This is a relatively high percentage, compared with teachers' usual practice.

Movement Patterns (Technique 13)

Another use of seating charts is to record the movements of teacher and students during a class lesson. We call this SCORE technique "movement patterns." The supervisor's task is to record how the teacher and individual students walk from one section of the room to another during a given time interval. This focus on *movement* differentiates movement patterns from the other SCORE techniques presented in this chapter: at task, which focuses on students' level of *attentiveness and engagement* in classroom tasks; and verbal flow, which focuses on the nature and direction of *verbal communication* in the classroom.

Many teaching situations, especially in primary and elementary school, require teachers to make decisions about where to position themselves in the classroom. For example, as students file into class after recess, the teacher needs to decide whether to stand by the door, at the desk, or elsewhere. When students are engaged in seatwork or group projects, the teacher must decide whether to stay at the desk or move around the room checking on students' work.

The nature of the teacher's movement patterns may affect classroom control and student attentiveness. The teacher who "hides" behind a desk may have more discipline problems than the teacher who checks on students as they work at their desks. The teacher who always stands in one position while speaking to the class may not hold students' attention as effectively as the teacher who moves about for dramatic emphasis or to illustrate a concept on the blackboard or chart.

Teachers may also reveal a consistent bias in their movement patterns. They may prefer one part of the classroom over another, perhaps because certain students are seated here. Some teachers consistently stand some distance away from students' seats while speaking to the class. This may create difficulties for students who do not see or hear well, and it may provide an excuse for some students to engage in off-task behavior ("the teacher can't see what I'm doing").

Students' movement patterns may reveal whether or not they are at task. Sometimes it is necessary for students to move about the classroom to complete an assigned activity. At other times students move about to avoid an assigned task or because they have no assigned task. The latter situation often occurs when students finish their work early in the class period; they mill around to find a classmate to engage in conversation or to find another activity.

Movement patterns can be recorded during any lesson, but the technique is most useful when the teaching situation contains the potential for movement about the classroom. For example, seatwork and group projects provide situations where the teacher needs to move about, and where students *do* move about even when they don't need to. On the other hand, the showing of a film or a question-and-answer recitation places many constraints on teacher and student movement. There is not likely to be much movement behavior to record.

Technique

The seating charts used in other SCORE instruments often consist of *interconnected* boxes, as in exhibit 7.1. To record movement patterns, each student and the teacher should be represented by *self-contained* boxes. Also, the seating chart should represent the physical layout of the classroom, including aisles and desks or tables where students might congregate.

Exhibits 7.4 and 7.5 show a seating chart used to record movement pattern data. Teacher or student movement from one point in the room to another is indicated by a continuous line. The line for each originates at the point where that person was located in the room when the supervisor began observing. The teacher and students are likely to move from one point to another, stop for a while, then move to another. Each stopping point should be represented by an indicator—for example, an arrow (——>——), a circle (——⊖——), or X (——X——). Exhibit 7.4 uses circled numbers to indicate stopping points. This physical movement chart shows that the teacher started the lesson standing at the front of the classroom, next moved to the student designated by box 1, and then proceeded to student 13.

A single line with a different symbol at each end can be used when a person goes from his desk to another location and then returns to his desk. For example, in exhibit 7.5 the teacher went from her desk (designated by O) to Wes's desk and then returned to her desk. In contrast, Keith went from his desk to the teacher's desk and then returned.

You may wish to indicate the pattern of movement at different points in the lesson. A supply of different colored pencils is useful for this purpose. For example, you might record the first ten minutes in yellow, the second ten minutes in green, and so on. If the teacher plans to divide the lesson into different activities, this can form the basis for color coding. The first activity might be direction giving, followed by small-group projects, followed by whole-class question-and-answer. Movement during each activity can be recorded with a different colored pencil. This technique helps the teacher analyze the pattern of movement that occurred at different stages of the lesson.

Occasionally so many students will mill about in the classroom that you will not be able to record all their movements. When this occurs, you may find it necessary to suspend data recording for a few minutes. (Make a note that you did so somewhere on your movement pattern chart.) Another possibility is to limit your observation to only certain students in the classroom.

Example

The movement pattern chart in exhibit 7.5 was recorded in a high school typing class. The teacher worried about whether he ran "too loose a ship." He didn't think that students should be "chained to their desks" during the entire class period, yet he wanted to instill in students a sense of discipline and self-control. He and the supervisor agreed that a movement pattern chart might be a good method for recording the extent of order-disorder in the classroom. The supervisor observed and recorded the class's movement behavior for approximately thirty minutes.

Data Analysis

At first glance a movement pattern chart such as the one shown in exhibit 7.5 looks like a hopeless maze. If teacher and supervisor isolate the behavior of one person or one section of the room, however, they usually can make helpful inferences from the chart.

The first thing that caught the teacher's eye was the door leading into the classroom. Six students entered or left the classroom after the lesson had begun. One student who was not enrolled in the class (indicated by a "?") apparently entered the classroom, talked to several friends and then left. The teacher thought that the mystery student probably was wandering about during his free study period. The chart also indicates that two other students (Bill and Sandra) entered late. Two students (Janice and Keith) left the class while it was in session and then returned. The teacher did not realize this had happened.

After inspecting these data, the teacher decided he needed to monitor students' entry and exit behavior more closely. Also included in this resolution to himself was the decision to give students some ground rules about leaving class while it is in session.

The teacher then focused his attention on his own movement

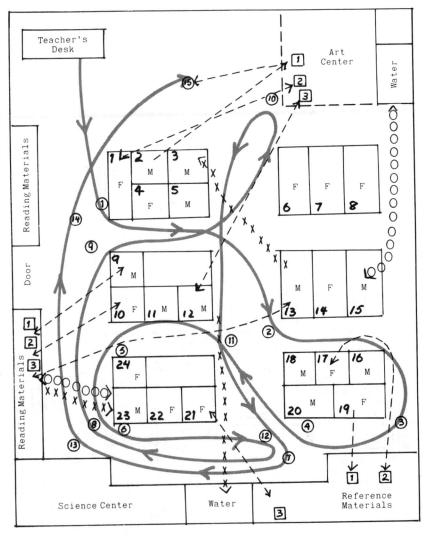

Physical Movement Legend

 X X X X X X X X X Directed student movement

— — — — — — — Purposeful student movement (nondirected)

▬▬▬▬▬▬ Teacher movement (arrow indicates direction)

O O O O O O Nonpurposeful student movement

① Student–teacher conference (number indicates sequential order)

Exhibit 7.4

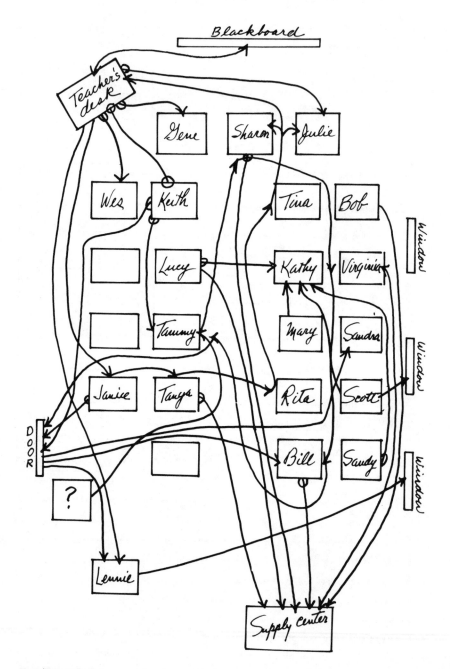

Exhibit 7.5. Movement pattern chart

behavior. He recalled that he had gone to the blackboard at the start of the lesson to write down key terms relating to typing business letters. Keith then came to his desk to ask a question. Next the teacher decided to check on students' progress, so he visited a few students (Lennie, Wes, Gene, and Julie), each time returning to his desk to catch up on some paperwork. Finally, he decided he should circulate a bit; this is reflected in the large loop starting and ending at his desk. Although he did not stop at every student's desk, he felt he got to each area of the classroom so that if a student desired to speak with him, the student could get his attention easily. The teacher generally felt satisfied with his movement pattern in this lesson.

He and the supervisor next turned their attention to the supply center. Six students (Tonya, Lucy, Sharon, Bill, Virginia, and Bob) went to the center for supplies during the observed part of the lesson. After seeing these data, the teacher wondered whether he should ask students to get any necessary materials at the start of the lesson. This procedure might create a more orderly class and might help students become more organized and systematic in their approach to typing. The supervisor suggested that the teacher experiment with this procedure and see for himself whether it produced the desired effects.

Finally, the teacher looked at other student behavior. He noted that several students had visited with each other, and in fact four of them (Lucy, Mary, Scott, and Sandy) had congregated around Kathy's desk. Two students (Scott and Lennie) had gone to the window to see what was happening outside. The supervisor told the teacher that most of this kind of classroom movement occurred near the end of the observation period. The teacher realized, then, that he had an activity planned for students who finished early but had forgotten to relay it to them because he was preoccupied about some paperwork he wanted to complete during the lesson.

Summing up his inferences from the movement chart data, the teacher felt that he might make a few changes that would create a more orderly class without losing the relaxed atmosphere he valued.

Notes

1. Frank McGraw, Jr., "The Use of 35-mm Time-Lapse Photography as a Feedback and Observation Instrument in Teacher Education" (Ann Arbor, MI: University Microfilms, No. 66–2516, 1966).
2. Gregg Jackson and Cecilia Cosca, "The Inequality of Educational Opportunity in the

Southwest: An Observational Study of Ethnically Mixed Classrooms," *American Educational Research Journal* 11 (1974): 219–29.
3. The report of the Jackson and Cosca study used the term "Anglo" to refer to white persons not of Spanish-speaking background. "Chicano" was used to refer to Mexican-Americans.
4. Ibid., p. 227.
5. Michael J. Dunkin and Bruce J. Biddle, *The Study of Teaching* (New York: Holt, Rinehart and Winston, 1974), p. 226.
6. Meredith D. Gall and Joyce P. Gall, "The Discussion Method," in *The Psychology of Teaching Methods*, ed. N. L. Gage (Chicago: National Society for the Study of Education, 1976).

8

Wide-Lens Techniques

"It was a shock to listen to the audiotape of my lesson. I never knew before how I sounded when talking to students. The idea of audiotaping lessons is good. After all, students have to hear you talk, so you might as well know how you sound to them. Just listening for a few minutes to the audiotape helped me learn quite a few things about how I communicate. I'm ready now to have myself videotaped. I want to see what that's like!"

—Comment of a preservice secondary teacher

Anecdotal Records (Technique 14)

The advantage of structured observation instruments such as at task, selective verbatim, and movement patterns is that they enable you to focus on a few classroom behaviors. Other classroom noise is screened out. But sometimes it is the "noise" (i.e., what you didn't plan to observe) that's most interesting. A particular teacher statement may strike you as especially good or bad or noteworthy. Possibly the teacher did something that made you think, "I wonder why she did that?"

Anecdotal records are a way to record classroom interaction using a wide lens. The basic technique is to make brief notes of events as they occur in the classroom. These notes form a "protocol" of what happened. Indeed, this is a favorite technique of anthropologists, who are highly trained in the process of making notes that objectively describe what happens in a different culture. The process of making intensive, direct observations is called *ethnography*.

The process of making good anecdotal records in supervisory observations is similar to the ethnographies anthropoligists make in observing the workings of different cultures. (Isn't the classroom a "culture"?) In fact, educational researchers are making increasing use of ethnographic methods to learn how classrooms function. For example, David Berliner and William Tikunoff employed ethnographers to record observations of classrooms known to vary in learning effectiveness.[1]

We use *anecdotal record* to describe this technique because it suggests informality and reminds teacher and supervisor that the record is not complete. Like any other classroom observation technique, the anecdotal record provides a selective set of data for the teacher to examine. Another reason for the label anecdotal record is that it is less esoteric than, say, ethnographic protocol, to which this technique is related.

Technique

The anecdotal record is a good technique to use when the teacher cannot think of specific behaviors that should be observed. This situation is most likely to occur in the beginning stages of supervision, that is, when the teacher is first learning about the planning conference–classroom observation–feedback conference cycle. The teacher may comment, "I guess I'd just like a general idea of what I'm like as a teacher." As supervisor, you might then suggest the anecdotal record as a broad-focus technique for collecting descriptive data about teacher and student behavior. Audio and video recordings, discussed later in this chapter, are other possibilities.

The anecdotal record is a broad-focus technique, but you and the teacher will need to decide just how wide to open the lens. You can make anecdotal observations of the teacher, one student, one group of students, the whole class of students, or everyone in the class (teacher, students, teacher aides, etc.). The wider the lens, the more behaviors can be observed. As you narrow the lens, you will have a narrower set of behaviors to observe, but you will also have the opportunity to make more intensive descriptions of these behaviors.

The anecdotal record usually consists of short descriptive sentences. Each sentence summarizes a discrete observation. You may wish to start each sentence on a separate line and every so often record the time that an observation was made. Thus the teacher can get a sense of the temporal flow of the events that occurred.

The sentences should be as objective and nonevaulative as

possible. Instead of writing "Students are bored," you might note "Several students yawn; Jane looks out window." Instead of writing "Teacher does good job of giving directions," you might note "Teacher gives clear directions. Asks if students understand. Most of class nod or say yes." If you make evaluative comments in your anecdotal record, the teacher is likely to react to the evaluation rather than to what occurred. If your comments are descriptive and neutral, the teacher can more easily form conclusions about the effectiveness of the lesson.

Teacher and student behaviors are not the only events to observe and describe in the anecdotal record. You should be alert also to the *context* of the teacher's lesson; for example:

"The room is warm; wall thermometer reads 78 degrees."
"Teacher shows map to class. Map is faded. Names of countries are difficult to read."
"Lesson is interrupted by announcement over intercom."
"One of the fluorescent lights starts to hum loudly."

An anecdotal record of these context events may help the teacher interpret certain behaviors of students (or of the teacher) that occurred during the lesson.

The anecdotal record consists of handwritten notes made by the supervisor as he or she sits unobtrusively somewhere in the classroom. Anthropologists often make handwritten ethnographic notes, too, but they have the option of using a portable audiotape recorder. As they make each observation, they simply make an audio-recorded description on the spot. This option is not usually available to a supervisor because he or she is physically too close to the teacher and students in the classroom.

Unless your handwriting is unusually legible, the anecdotal record will be difficult for the teacher to read and study. The preferred practice is to have your notes typed so that the teacher has a neat typed transcript to reflect on in the feedback conference. Also, a typed transcript has a more objective, neutral appearance than a set of handwritten notes.

Example

Exhibit 8.1 presents a sample of an ethnographic protocol made by a professionally trained ethnographer.[2] It represents the rich description possible with this method. Anecdotal records made by clinical

Protocol Number: 06
Name of Researcher: Gail
Date of Observation:
Subject of Observation:

2nd Grade Class, Open

1. Classroom, with two team teacher
2. and two other adults.
3. This is a joint observation with
4. Elizabeth. I will be observing two
5. reading groups today, simultan-
6. eously, including 9 children. Out of
7. the nine children, 2 are girls, 7 are
8. boys.

8:30 Noise level 2

10. At 8:30 the noise level is 2. The
11. children have just been let into the
12. classroom, taking their coats off
13. and wandering around the room.
14. Several boys are in the corner
15. fighting, and some girls are sitting
16. on the floor playing a puzzle. The
17. teacher is walking back and forth in
18. the back of the classroom not at-
19. tending the children. The noise
20. continues and the children are run-
21. ning around. There is much con-
22. fusion in the room. Two teachers

8:35 23. stand at the desk talking to one
24. another. At 8:35, Mrs. Tyler
25. leaves the room. The team teach-
26. er stays seated behind the class-
27. room at her desk. At 8:40 Mrs.

28. Tyler comes back into the room.
29. She walks to the desk at the far
30. left hand side of the classroom,
31. which is a round table, and sits
32. on the edge. She says "Blue
33. Group, get your folders and go up
34. in the front. Green Group, come
35. here." Noise levels drop to 1, and
36. the children begin to follow her
37. orders. She says, "Anybody lose
38. a quarter?" No one responds, and
39. she repeats the question again
40. with irritation in her voice. She
41. says I know someone found.
42. someone lost a quarter because
43. it was found in the coat room.
44. Look in your pockets and see."
45. No one says anything.
46. She now stands up and pulls a
47. pile of workbooks from across
48. the table over to her. They are
49. the   reading workbooks.
50. She opens one of them on the
51. top and says, "Ah Daniel!" She
52. says this with a loud sharp voice.
53. She continues, "Your work yes-
54. terday was not too bad but you
55. need some work. Evidently there
56. are still some words you don't
57. understand." She thumbs through
58. the rest of his lesson. Danny is
59. standing at the outside of the cir-
60. cle around her, not listening to

61. what she is saying, Mrs. Tyler
62. now stands and gives instructions
63. to the Green Group. She tells
64. them to go through 8 through 13,
65. reading the two stories between
66. those pages and to go over the
67. work in the workbooks that she is
68. about to give back. She tells them
69. that they may seat any place but
70. not together and she says, "And I
71. don't want any funny business."
72. She now opens the next work-
73. book which is Nicole's. She tells
74. Nicole that she is having the
75. same problem that Danny is hav-
76. ing without specifying further.
77. Nicole looks up at her with an ex-
78. pectant look on her face. She
79. then looks at a third book and
80. says "Michelle, you're having the
81. same problem." She says,
82. "Snatch means to grab. Beach.
83. what does it mean?" Michelle
84. doesn't answer. She has her fin-
85. ger in her mouth and looks anx-
86. ious. The teacher closes the
87. workbook and pushes it to
88. Michelle. Michelle takes it and
89. walks away. with Nicole. Teacher
90. then opens the next workbook
91. and says. "Mike, I don't appreci-
92. ate all these circles. She points

Exhibit 8.1. A sample protocol

supervisors do not usually have the same amount of detail, although this is possible if the supervisor becomes proficient in quick note taking.

You might observe in exhibit 8.1 that the ethnographer does not focus on a particular child or a particular category of teacher behavior. The ethnographer instead records any salient event as it occurs. In this particular protocol the salient events seem to relate to the teacher's management and direction-giving techniques. The teacher can review the protocol to determine whether she wishes to maintain or change these techniques.

Video and Audio Recordings (Technique 15)

Video and audio recordings are probably the most objective observation techniques. They allow teachers to see themselves as students see them. Another advantage of recordings is that they have a wide focus. They can pick up a great deal of what teachers and students are doing and saying. A good recording captures the "feel" of classroom interaction.

Video and audio recorders are becoming increasingly accessible as supervision tools. Not too many years ago these devices were expensive and bulky. Their cost, especially the cost of audio recorders, is now well within the reach of educational institutions. Unfortunately, video and audio recorders are used infrequently in teacher supervision even when the equipment is available. Video recorders are much more likely to be used in the coaching of school sports. Athletes and their coaches spend hours analyzing films or video recordings of games and individual player actions. Shouldn't we spend a fraction of our supervisory time with teachers reviewing recordings of their classroom interaction?

The portable video recorder is an integral component of the microteaching method.[3] Microteaching, which was developed at Stanford University in the 1960s, is widely considered to be an important innovation in the training of teachers. In microteaching the teacher practices a few specific teaching skills in a scaled-down teaching situation involving a ten- or fifteen-minute lesson with five or so students. The microteaching lesson is videotaped and played back to the teacher so that his or her teaching performance, especially the use of target skills, can be analyzed.

Teachers almost invariably find that the video recording provides an important self-learning experience. Nevertheless, there are several problems to avoid. First, supervisors must be careful to arrange the video recording equipment so that it does not interfere with the lesson. This is best done by setting up the equipment ahead of time, before students enter the classroom. Second, our experience indicates that teachers, when first exposed to a videotape of themselves, tend to focus on the "cosmetics" of their performance (e.g., physical appearance, clothes, and voice quality). In fact, a study by Gavrial Salomon and Fred McDonald revealed that in a videotape replay situation, 58 percent of teachers' self-observations were concerned with physical appearance, and only 18 percent were focused on teaching behavior.[4] This is a natural reaction. Ways to deal with it are suggested later in this section.

Another problem is that some teachers initially are anxious about the prospect of being videotaped. This problem can be alleviated by allowing teachers to experiment with the equipment before the classroom lesson is to be videotaped. Another helpful procedure is to allow a teacher to keep his or her own videotape or show the teacher how to erase the video recording. This calms any fear that the video recording might get into the "wrong" hands.

Although video recordings would seem to be a more powerful observational tool than audio recordings, this may not be so. Teachers sometimes are captivated by the image on the TV screen and do not listen to what is being said. Audio recordings have fewer distracting cues, and so it is easier for the teacher to concentrate on the verbal interaction. Research has shown that video and audio feedback are equally effective in helping teachers improve their use of verbal teaching skills.[5]

Technique

The first step in making audio or video recordings is to obtain equipment that is in good working order. The portable video recorder typically includes (1) a TV camera; (2) a microphone; (3) a videotape recorder (VTR), which looks something like a reel-to-reel audio recorder; (4) a viewing screen, which looks like a regular TV set; and (5) wires for connecting the various components of the system. In addition, a supply of videotapes and a videotape pickup reel are needed.

Because video recorders are relatively difficult to set up and dismantle, we suggest that you find a free room where the equipment can be used and stored, especially if more than one teacher's classroom is to be videotaped. Each teacher can bring his or her class to this room, conduct the lesson, and then return to the teacher's regular classroom. Perhaps later the same day the teacher can return to the taping room and view the videotape replay.

Audio recorders are much simpler to set up and operate. Many self-contained models include a built-in microphone and operate on batteries. These recorders usually are designed for audio cassettes, which contain the audiotape and pickup reel in a small enclosed unit.

The recording process becomes more complicated as the size of the class increases. It is much easier to video-record or audio-record a group of five students than a group of thirty students. Most microphones for audio and video recorders have a small pickup range. As the focus of supervision is usually the teacher, we suggest that you place the microphone fairly close to the teacher. By doing so, you are likely to record everything the teacher says and some of what students say.

Teachers can learn to make their own video recordings, but in many situations it is more helpful if you, the supervisor, are present to make the recording. You need to find a convenient place to set up the camera on a stationary base; then, change the lens focus and turn the camera to follow the teacher as the lesson proceeds. Some systems allow you to "handhold" the camera so that you can walk around the classroom and make close-up recordings of events that interest you or the teacher.

A thirty-minute recording is usually more than adequate. It will try the teacher's patience and yours to play back a recording that is any longer than this. One procedure you can use is to have the teacher play back the entire recording for himself. He can share insights about his teaching performance with you during the feedback conference. At this time you can select a short segment of the recording (perhaps three to five minutes) for more intensive analysis. You will find that even a brief segment can yield many insights into the teacher's skill level and teaching style.

The wide focus of video or audio recordings is both a strength and a weakness. The insightful teacher will be able to observe many different aspects of teacher behavior and student behavior. Some teachers will notice only a few aspects, however, and may focus on the "cosmetic" features mentioned earlier. Your role in the feedback conference is to guide the teacher's observations, encouraging the teacher to draw inferences whenever possible, but also drawing the teacher's attention to significant classroom phenomena if they are being overlooked.

Example

Teaching Strategies is a required course in the secondary education program at the University of Oregon. Similar course content is part of teacher-education programs in many other colleges and universities. In Teaching Strategies students are asked to attend microteaching sessions in which they practice several different teaching methods. Students audio-record their lessons for later analysis. They also are required to make a transcript covering several minutes of the audio recording. This procedure ensures that students listen very carefully to what was said.

Exhibit 8.2 presents a partial transcript made by a student who had done a poetry lesson using the lecture method. This example shows that an audio recording and transcript made from it provided a rich source of feedback to the student on his teaching behavior.

Students in the Teaching Strategies course are also asked to write an analysis of their lesson based on the transcript and other feedback data. Exhibit 8.3 presents the first part of an analysis written by the student who gave the poetry lesson. It illustrates that the process of teaching a lesson and audio-recording it for later analysis is a powerful technique for helping the student see areas for instructional improvement.

Preservice teachers, including the one discussed here, tend to criticize themselves too severely in their initial encounters with self-audio recording. The supervisor can ameliorate this problem by reassuring students that flaws noted in their teaching performance are commonplace and can be eliminated with practice.

Notes

1. David C. Berliner and William J. Tikunoff, "The California Beginning Teacher Evaluation Study: Overview of the Ethnographic Study," *Journal of Teacher Education* 27 (1976): 24–30.
2. Ibid., p. 25.
3. Dwight W. Allen and Kevin Ryan, *Microteaching* (Reading, MA: Addison-Wesley, 1969).
4. Gavrial Salomon and Fred J. McDonald, "Pre- and Posttest Reactions to Self-Viewing One's Performance on Videotape" (paper presented at the annual meeting of the American Psychological Association, 1968).
5. Meredith D. Gall et al., "Improving Teachers' Mathematics Tutoring Skills Through Microteaching: A Comparison of Videotape and Audiotape Feedback" (paper presented at the annual meeting of the American Educational Research Association, 1971).

Interesting

CI 314

0:00	OK, um, what I want to talk about is, uh, a poem by Denise Levertov, called "Living." (pause) And the reason I wanted to talk about this is because I think it's something that I can cover in 10 minutes, and uh, well, not in, not entirely but it's short enough to go over the basics, and, uh, Denise Levertov I, I think is, is . . . one of the
0:30	greatest of living poets, and not, not as well known as she should be. This poem in particular I think is, is, uh, one of her greatest poems, and it's not as well known as many, many poems that aren't nearly as good. (pause) Um, what I want to do is, is, is approach the poem in
1:00	terms of how it's organized . . . 'cause that's one way to get a grip, a grasp on a poem and Uh, not so much talk about what it says as, as the way it's, the way it's set up, um, and I, I don't think that's the only way to read a poem, in fact I don't think it's a very complete way but it's, um, it can lead you farther into a poem sometimes than
1:30	just talking about what it's about. And so let me just start with the way it sounds to me: "The fire in leaf and grass/ so green it seems/ each summer the last summer.// The wind blowing, the leaves/ shivering in the sun,/ each day the last day.// A red salamander/ so cold and so/ easy to catch, dreamily// moves his delicate feet/ and long tail. I hold/ my hand open for him to go.// Each minute the last minute."
2:00	(Pause) OK, um, it seems to me that that poem holds together very well. It's, it's a very tightly knit poem. Um. But it's not held together in any of the, the traditional ways: it's not, it doesn't have a rhyme scheme, there's no beat or rhythm that carries you along.
2:30	And so if you look at it – Well, does everybody agree that, it doesn't, it doesn't seem like a fragmented poem? It goes, it goes along, and I think it builds, builds very strongly towards its conclusion. Um . . . to start with, to start with the smallest units, just to
3:00	look at the sounds of the poem, and the way it . . . the way the sounds hold together – Starting in the first line: the, the first significant word is "fire." And you see that the "f" sound is repeated immediately in "leaf." And the "r" sound in "fire" carries forward into "grass," which then carries you forward into "green" again, and then down to the
3:30	"r" ending in "summer" and "summer" which is repeated. And then you see these, the "r" sound particularly you find again down in the poem down in the the uh, in "shivering" which repeats the "er" sound from "summer"--and that turns up again in "salamander" in the last, next to last triplet. And then the, when you get into "leaf" the, the
4:00	"ea" sound from "leaf" is repeated twice in the next line in "green" and in "seems"--and in "each" and in "leaves" in the next, the next stanza, and then, then you hear it again in "each"--in "easy"--in "dreamily"--in "feet"--and then again in "each" in the last line.
4:30	(Pause) And, um . . . these, these sounds (pause) are, um--well, the, uh, the tying together of the, of the poem through the, through the, uh, the sounds in the words goes on throughout the poem. For instance: if you look for the "o" sound, you don't see it until you get into the poem, but it turns up towards the end. If you move down
5:00	toward, to the third verse, it starts coming in very strongly, in this in a line "so cold and so/ easy to catch"--then it turns up again in "I hold my hand open for him to go." And these, these are, these are, these are the significant sounds in the poem. And this, this technique that Levertov relies on very, very strongly in a lot
5:30	of her writing is called "assonance." Um, I--does, everyone know what the meaning of assonance is? There's, there's two, uh, basic techniques used, but a lot of modern poets--assonance

Exhibit 8.2. Transcript of lecture micro-lesson (October 7, 1976)

It wasn't a disaster. I think the students in the group and I learned some things about poetry from it. ↓

I would rate this lecture <u>as a disaster</u>, and this
for two main reasons which are not unrelated:
nervousness and poor organization. A sudden attack
of stage fright was for some reason quite
unexpected, and because I hadn't anticipated it I
hadn't written out any more than a general outline
of the points I wanted to cover. This, as it turned
out, was not enough to see me through. Some of the
faults in this lecture, such as the astonishing
number of "um's," "uh's," and stuttering repetitions
(e.g., "What I want to do is, is, is approach the
poem . . .") are simply signs of nervous excitement;
having heard tapes of myself in conversation, I know
these mannerisms are not always present, at least
not to this degree. These I can only expect to
correct by calming down a bit, but this I think I
will be able to do if I correct some of the more
fundamental mistakes I made this time around.
  The most important thing missing from this lecture
is an introduction. Immediately upon hearing the
first questions after I finished, I was made aware
that I had left out the necessary background for
reading the poem. And even though biographical
information about the author, for instance, was not
what I was mainly concerned with, it would have
given students <u>some</u> context, which is a necessary
preliminary to any appreciation. A preliminary
statement of what the poem is <u>about, or perhaps
simply some lead-in remarks about summer days and
why some moments seem more alive than others, would
have been very useful.</u> And although before the
lecture I had wanted not to seem too schematic,
afterwards I realized that I needn't have worried:
and I now regret not having outlined ahead of time
the areas I was going to cover.

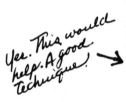

Yes. This would help. A good technique. →

  It now seems to me, also, that I went at the poem
exactly backwards: for some reason I began with the
smallest details, the sounds of the poem, and went
on to its larger structure before talking about its
over-all theme. This is absolutely perverse; it is
almost as if I had been trying to keep the main point
a secret until the last possible moment. Clearly, it
would have been better to begin with the most
general statements, and to proceed to the more
particular ones only after these landmarks had been
mapped out.
  I feel that, even so, using a blackboard would have
improved things immeasurably. Not only could I have
communicated better by writing down a few terms like
"assonance" and by marking the repetitions of sounds
rather than simply listing them; but also I think it
would have helped simply to get everyone's eyes and
attention (not least of all my own) away from the
handout sheet <u>and out into a more central meeting
place.</u> I even think that just having something to do
with my hands would have put me more at ease.

nice phrase →

  I only asked questions twice in the course of the
lecture, and both questions were almost rhetorical,
being put in such a way as to actually discourage a
response: the first one beginning "does everyone

agree . . ." and the second one beginning "does
everyone know . . ." There were several other places
in the lecture where a question would have been in
order: and all of the questions should have been
less leading, more open to genuine answers. This
constricted questioning is, again, at least partly a
function of nervousness; as is the fact that I
forgot to ask for questions at the end.

Exhibit 8.3. Lecture micro-lesson evaluation

9

Checklists and Timeline Coding

"The man who can make a hard thing easy is the educator."
—Emerson

The observation instruments described in the previous chapters are relatively unstructured. In using selective verbatim, the SCORE techniques, anecdotal records, or video and audio recordings, teacher and supervisor jointly decide the categories of behavior to be observed. Occasionally, as a supervisor, you may wish to use a more highly structured instrument to observe behavior. You may prefer such instruments, or perhaps a particular instrument is well suited for your immediate purpose.

In chapter 3 we presented several checklists that teachers self-administer to identify their concerns about teaching. Now we present checklists that students complete to give feedback to their teachers, and checklists that the supervisor completes while observing a teacher's classroom behavior.[1] In addition, we describe a special checklist procedure called "timeline coding" that is useful for detecting patterns in classroom events.

Student-Administered Checklists

As students participate in class, they have the opportunity to make extensive observations of their teacher's behavior. Summaries of students' observations can be useful in clinical supervision because teachers often are very concerned about how their students perceive them (even more than they are concerned about how supervisors perceive them!).

Teacher Image Questionnaire (Technique 16)

The Teacher Image Questionnaire (TIQ) was developed by Roy C. Bryan for administration to junior high and high school students. A copy of the TIQ form is presented in exhibit 9.1. Students are invited to list "strengths of your teacher" and "weaknesses of your teacher" on the back side of the form.

Administration of the TIQ requires about fifteen minutes. The data can be summarized in various ways. Perhaps the simplest procedure is to calculate the percentage of students who check each point (e.g., "poor," "excellent") for each questionnaire item. For a nominal fee, a scoring service will analyze the response sheets and prepare a report for the teacher.[2]

A study by Bryan indicated that the majority of teachers change their teaching behavior after studying their TIQ profiles.[3] In another study, he found that student ratings of teachers generally agreed with administrator ratings of the same teachers.[4]

Pupil Observation Survey (Technique 17)

The Pupil Observation Survey is a student-administered checklist that measures five different dimensions of teacher performance.[5] These dimensions reflect the extent to which the teacher

1. Is friendly, cheerful, admired
2. Is knowledgable, poised
3. Is interesting, preferred to other teachers
4. Uses strict control
5. Uses democratic procedure

The thirty-eight items of the Pupil Observation Survey can be used by students grade five and higher. If you wish to use a short version of this checklist, the Student Evaluation of Teaching form is available. A copy of it is presented in exhibit 9.2.

Prepared by Educator Feedback Center, Western Michigan University, Kalamazoo, Michigan 49008

TEACHER-IMAGE QUESTIONNAIRE

USE LEAD PENCIL.

Do not b᾽   ᾽til you are told to do so by the person in charge.

WHAT IS YOU.   'ON CONCERNING THIS TEACHER'S:

	POOR	FAIR	AVERAGE	GOOD	EXCELLENT

1. KNOWLEDGΕ   ᾽JECT: (Does he have a thorough knowledge and understanding   ᾽aching field?) — POOR FAIR AVG GOOD EXC

2. CLARITY OF PRESE.   ᾽N: (Are ideas presented at a level which you can understand?) — POOR FAIR AVG GOOD EXC

3. FAIRNESS: (Is he fair ar.   ᾽tial in his treatment of all students in the class?) — POOR FAIR AVG GOOD EXC

4. CONTROL: (Is the classroom ι   ᾽but also relaxed and friendly?) — POOR FAIR AVG GOOD EXC

5. ATTITUDE TOWARD STUDENTS: (ι   feel that this teacher likes you?) — POOR FAIR AVG GOOD EXC

6. SUCCESS IN STIMULATING INTEREST: ι   class interesting and challenging?) — POOR FAIR AVG GOOD EXC

7. ENTHUSIASM: (Does he show interest in a   ᾽husiasm for the subject? Does he appear to enjoy teaching this   ?) — POOR FAIR AVG GOOD EXC

8. ATTITUDE TOWARD STUDENT IDEAS: (Does this teͺ   ᾽ve respect for the things you have to say in class?) — POOR FAIR AVG GOOD EXC

9. ENCOURAGEMENT OF STUDENT PARTICIPATION: (Doeͺ   ᾽acher encourage you to raise questions and express ideas in cͺ — POOR FAIR AVG GOOD EXC

10. SENSE OF HUMOR: (Does he share amusing experiences and ᴵͺ   ᾽ his own mistakes?) — POOR FAIR AVG GOOD EXC

11. ASSIGNMENTS: (Are assignments sufficiently challenging withͺ   ᾽OR FAIR AVG GOOD EXC being unreasonably long?)

12. APPEARANCE: (Are his grooming and dress in good taste?) — ᾽R AVG GOOD EXC

13. OPENNESS: (Is this teacher able to see things from your point of view?) — POOR   ᾽ GOOD EXC

14. SELF-CONTROL: (Does this teacher become angry when little problems arise in the classroom?) — POOR FAIR   ᾽ EXC

15. CONSIDERATION OF OTHERS: (Is he patient, understanding, considerate, and courteous?) — POOR FAIR AVG ᴳ

16. EFFECTIVENESS: (What is your overall evaluation of your teacher's effectiveness?) — POOR FAIR AVG GOOD Ε

OVER

Form TIQ-0969

Exhibit 9.1

STUDENT EVALUATION OF TEACHING

D. J. VELDMAN and R. F. PECK

TEACHER'S LAST NAME: _____

SUBJECT: _____

SCHOOL: _____

CIRCLE THE RIGHT CHOICES BELOW

Teacher's Sex: M   F

My Sex: M   F

My Grade Level:

3   4   5   6   7   8   9   10   11   12

DO NOT USE

CIRCLE <u>ONE</u> OF THE FOUR CHOICES IN FRONT OF EACH STATEMENT.
THE FOUR CHOICES MEAN:

F = Very Much False
f = More False Than True
t = More True Than False
T = Very Much True

This Teacher:

F f t T   is always friendly toward students.

F f t T   knows a lot about the subject.

F f t T   is never dull or boring.

F f t T   expects a lot from students.

F f t T   asks for students' opinions before making decisions.

F f t T   is usually cheerful and optimistic.

F f t T   is not confused by unexpected questions.

F f t T   makes learning more like fun than work.

F f t T   doesn't let students get away with anything.

F f t T   often gives students a choice in assignments.

Exhibit 9.2

Student Perception of Teacher Style (Technique 18)

The Student Perception of Teacher Style (SPOTS) is a checklist that measures students' perceptions about their teacher's level of directiveness.[6] The seventeen items of the checklist measure the extent to which the teacher uses the following directive behaviors:

1. Formal planning and structuring of coursework
2. Minimization of informal work or small-group work
3. Rigid structuring of such small-group work as it is employed
4. Rigid structuring of individual and class activities
5. Emphasis on factual knowledge or knowledge derived from sources of authority
6. Use of absolute and justifiable punishment
7. Minimization of opportunities for students to make and learn from mistakes
8. Maintenance of formal relationship with students
9. Assumption of total responsibility for grades
10. Maintenance of formal classroom atmosphere

The complete checklist is presented in exhibit 9.3.

Although SPOTS was originally validated with eleventh- and twelfth-grade students, it also should be suitable for administration to younger students.

Observer-Administered Checklists

As a clinical supervisor, you may choose to construct your own checklist for recording observations of classroom behavior. Here are several checklists we have constructed for our own use in supervision. You are invited to use them as is or to adapt them to your particular purpose.

Question-and-Answer Teaching (Technique 19)

Question asking sometimes occurs when the teacher is introducing a new topic, but it is most often used to review curriculum materials students have just finished reading or seeing. For example, question asking may occur after students have read a chapter in a book, seen a

1. Your teacher is mainly interested in

1	2	3	4	5	6	7	8	9

How many facts you know	If he gets an idea across to you	Whether you can "think" for yourself

2. The teacher

1	2	3	4	5	6	7	8	9

Makes you do what he wants you to most of the time	Makes you do what he wants you to sometimes	Lets you make your own decisions most of the time

3. The teacher

1	2	3	4	5	6	7	8	9

Doesn't like to talk about any subject that isn't part of your course	Talks about your course subject a lot but encourages the discussion of other matters	Likes to talk about different subjects and is interested in your personal opinions

4. The students in our class

1	2	3	4	5	6	7	8	9

Only speak when the teacher asks them a question	Feel free to ask the teacher questions	Feel free to speak up at almost any time

5. When the teacher or another student says something you don't agree with

1	2	3	4	5	6	7	8	9

You try not to start an argument and feel that it's not your job to tell him he's wrong	You tell him why you disagree when the teacher asks you to	You feel free to discuss and argue your point of view whether the teacher asks you or not

6. The teacher

1	2	3	4	5	6	7	8	9

Usually bases his opinions on what the book says or what the principal says	Usually gives you another point of view in addition to what the book says	Tells you that books, teachers, principals and customs are not always right

7. If you were to call your teacher by his first name,

1	2	3	4	5	6	7	8	9

He wouldn't like it and would tell you not to do it	He would tell you that it's alright to call him by his first name outside of school but that he would prefer you to call him by his last name while he is teaching	He wouldn't mind at all

8. The teacher

1	2	3	4	5	6	7	8	9

Never tells jokes while he's teaching and does not like it when the students joke around	Sometimes tells a joke or a humorous story to get a point across	Always tells funny stories and encourages the students to tell about funny things that have happened to them

9. The teacher spends a lot of time

1	2	3	4	5	6	7	8	9

Telling you about tests, grades and about how the course is planned	Giving you an idea about tests, grades and the course but not too much time giving you the details	Asking you to make your own decisions about tests, grades, the course plan or group projects

10. When we are working on a group project or in a committee, the teacher

1   2   3   4   5   6 7   8   9

Tells us exactly what to do	Suggests ways that the project might be handled	Lets the group members decide how the project should be handled

11. The teacher usually

1   2   3   4   5   6 7   8   9

Makes all the students do the same thing in class (working, studying)	Makes some students work on projects and some students study, depending on how far behind they are	Lets the students do what they like as long as they complete the number of projects or chapters assigned by the end of the week .

12. When you get angry at the teacher,

1   2   3   4   5   6 7   8   9

You usually hold it in because the teacher would punish any show of anger	You feel that you can tell the teacher why you're angry	You feel that you could show your anger without the teacher becoming angry

13. The teacher

1   2   3   4   5   6 7   8   9

Acts like a teacher all of the time	Acts like a teacher most of the time but sometimes seems more like a friend	Acts like a friend more than he acts like a teacher

14. The first thing the teacher does when he comes into the room

1   2   3   4   5   6 7   8   9

Is to tell you to be quiet so that he can take attendance	Is to take attendance and ask you why some students are absent (if they are sick, etc.)	Is to let you start your projects or studying and then takes attendance while you're working

15. In this class homework

1   •   2   3   4   5   6 7   8   9

Is assigned every day and must be handed in the next day	Is divided between work which is due every day and a few long term projects each term	Usually consists of long-term projects

16. In our class pupils work together in a group or on a committee

1   2   3   4   5   6 7   8   9

Never	Sometimes	A great deal

17. When there is work which has to be done with another student we are

1   2   3   4   5   6 7   8   9

Usually told with whom to work	Can sometimes choose our own work partner	Can usually decide with whom we want to work

Exhibit 9.3. Student perception of teacher style (revised) (SPOTS)

film, completed a science experiment, or participated in a role-playing exercise.

The Question-and-Answer Checklist shown in exhibit 9.4 is organized around three types of behaviors. First are teacher behaviors that often lead to increased student participation in the lesson. Research shows that, unless teachers have received special training, they are likely to dominate the lesson by speaking two thirds of the time. One technique to increase student participation is to call on nonvolunteers to respond. Teachers are likely to call on students who raise their hands and who customarily give good answers to their questions. Yet nonvolunteers often make good contributions if the teacher takes the initiative by calling on them.

Student participation also can be increased by redirecting the same question to several students. The teacher may invite additional responses to a question by a nod acknowledging a particular student or by a statement such as "Does anyone have a different idea?" or "Would someone like to add to what Susie said?" Praising answers is a technique that helps students feel that their answers are worthwhile; as a result, they are encouraged to speak up when other questions are asked. Another good technique is to ask students if they have any questions of their own about the lesson content. The teacher may choose to answer these student-initiated questions directly or may call on other students to answer them.

The second category in the Question-and-Answer Checklist refers

Behaviors That Increase Student Participation
1. Calls on nonvolunteers
2. Redirects question
3. Praises student responses
4. Invites student-initiated questions

Behaviors That Elicit Thoughtful Responses
1. Asks higher cognitive questions
2. Pauses 3-5 seconds after asking a question
3. Asks follow-up questions to an initial response

Negative Behaviors
1. Reacts negatively to student response
2. Repeats own question
3. Asks multiple questions
4. Answers own questions
5. Repeats student's answer

Strong Points of Lesson

Suggestions for Improvement

Exhibit 9.4. Checklist for question-and-answer teaching

to the cognitive level of the teacher's lesson. Educators generally agree that students should not just recite back the facts they have learned. (This is done by asking simple fact questions of the Who, What, Where, When variety.) Students also should be encouraged to *think* about the curriculum content. This goal is accomplished by asking higher cognitive questions, which are questions that cannot be answered simply by looking in the textbook. The student must think and formulate an original response. Higher cognitive questions may ask the student to compare and contrast, state possible motives or causes for observed phenomena, draw conclusions, provide evidence, make predictions, solve problems, make judgments, or offer opinions.

Asking a higher cognitive question may not be sufficient to elicit a thoughtful response. One helpful behavior is to pause several seconds before calling on a student to respond.[7] This gives students time to think. It also encourages all students in the class to generate an answer because they do not know whom the teacher will call on to respond.

The third technique for eliciting thoughtful responses on the checklist is to ask follow-up questions after the student has given an initial answer to a question. For example, the teacher might ask, "Did you agree with the jury's verdict?" and the student might respond, "No, I didn't." The teacher can follow up by asking the student to support his position (e.g., "Why didn't you agree?"). Follow-up questions also can be used to encourage a student to clarify a vague answer (e.g., "I'm not sure I understood what you said. Can you restate your answer?"), to generate additional ideas (e.g., "Can you think of other ways of solving the energy crisis?"), or to challenge the student (e.g., "That's a good idea, but have you considered possible adverse consequences that might occur if your idea was put into practice?"). Follow-up questions can be used, too, to prompt a student who is unable to respond to the initial question.

The first two categories of behavior in the checklist in exhibit 9.4 refer to the "do's" of question asking. The third category refers to the "don'ts." Teachers should avoid reacting negatively to student responses by making critical remarks (e.g., "That doesn't make any sense at all") or by showing annoyance. Critical behavior only increases the likelihood that the student will volunteer no response in the future. The second negative behavior, repeating one's question, is to be avoided because it wastes class time and encourages students not to listen carefully the first time the teacher asks a particular question. The third "don't," asking multiple questions, refers to the practice of asking several questions in a row before settling on a question to which a response is invited. Teachers tend to do this when they are unsure of the lesson content or if they are inclined to think aloud. Multiple questions also waste class time, and they are likely to confuse students.

The final "don't" is repeating student answers verbatim. A better practice is to praise the answer, extend the answer by adding new information, or invite another student to build on the answer.

The bottom two headings of the checklist provide an open-ended opportunity for the observer to comment on strong points of the lesson and areas in which the teacher may need to improve.

Lecture-Explanation Teaching (Technique 20)

As we have pointed out, research indicates that the average teacher does two thirds of the talking in the elementary and secondary classroom.[8] The percentage is probably higher in some settings (e.g., college teaching) and lower in others. Much of this "talk time" is spent in presenting new concepts and information to students, or in explaining difficult parts of the curriculum. We have found that many teachers say they rarely use lecture as a teaching strategy when, in fact, much of their time is spent talking to students—presenting new curriculum content or explaining ideas and procedures.

The checklist shown in exhibit 9.5 is designed for analyzing various aspects of the teacher's lecture-explanation behavior. You will note that the checklist is in two parts. The first part includes behaviors that can be tallied each time they occur. The tallies are counted to determine how often the teacher used a particular lecture-explanation behavior during the lesson. Some of these behaviors are techniques for increasing the meaningfulness of the curriculum content—for example, the technique of giving examples to illustrate a concept. Other behaviors are techniques for involving students so that they do not sit passively through the entire lecture-explanation. Asking students if they have questions about the lesson is an example of a technique that usually creates student involvement.

The second part of the checklist is a list of teacher behaviors rated by the observer. Some of the rated behaviors concern how well the teacher organizes the lecture content. For example, repeating key points and summarizing them at the end of the lesson is a technique that helps students organize the various ideas in the lecture as "more important" or "less important."

BEHAVIORS TO BE TALLIED

Meaningful Content
1. Relates lecture content to content already familiar to students
2. Gives example to illustrate concept
3. Gives explanation for generalization or opinion

Student Involvement
1. Asks students if they have questions
2. Directs question to students
3. Has students engage in activity

BEHAVIORS TO BE RATED

Organization	good	needs improve- ment
1. Lecture has clear organization and sequence		5 4 3 2 1
2. Uses blackboard, handout, etc., to show organization of lecture	5 4 3 2 1	
3. Tells students what (s)he expects students to remember from lecture		5 4 3 2 1
4. Repeats key points and summarizes them at end	5 4 3 2 1	
5. Avoids digressions		5 4 3 2 1

Delivery	good	needs improve- ment
1. Speaks slowly and clearly		5 4 3 2 1
2. Conveys enthusiasm		5 4 3 2 1
3. Avoids reading from lecture notes		5 4 3 2 1
4. Avoids filler phrases such as "you know"		5 4 3 2 1
5. Avoids nervous gestures		5 4 3 2 1
6. Maintains eye contact with students		5 4 3 2 1
7. Uses humor		5 4 3 2 1

Exhibit 9.5. Checklist for lecture-explanation teaching

The largest category of behaviors in the checklist relates to the teacher's skill in delivery. Lecture-explanation uses speech as its medium, and so the teacher's mastery of oral delivery determines in large part how well the curriculum content is conveyed to students. The enthusiasm in the teacher's voice, the clarity of the teacher's remarks, the avoidance of nervous gestures and filler phrases—all contribute to the overall effectiveness of the lesson.

As in the Question-and-Answer Checklist (exhibit 9.4), this checklist can be augmented by including space for additional comments about the strong points of the lesson and suggestions for improvement.

Other Checklists

We have presented two checklists for observing two general strategies of teaching—question-and-answer and lecture-explanation. Other checklists are available for observing more specific teaching strategies. For example, Bruce Joyce and his colleagues present rating checklists for observing teaching strategies organized into three models: information processing, social interaction, and personal.[9]

Flanders Interaction Analysis

The best-known technique for classroom observation is the Flanders Interaction Analysis System.[10] This technique has been extensively researched and is widely used in teacher-training programs. It is called Interaction Analysis because the observation categories are used to record all verbal interactions that occur between teacher and students in a classroom setting. The record is analyzed to determine the verbal patterns that characterize the teaching style used by the teacher.

Our discussion of this technique is intended to familiarize you with its use in teacher supervision. Several excellent materials are available to help you acquire skills for using Interaction Analysis to make classroom observations.[11] It would certainly be worth your time to learn this technique in depth. We believe that you and the teachers under your supervision will find that it is a powerful tool for analyzing the act of teaching.

The Flanders Interaction Analysis System has two principal features: (1) verbal interaction categories, and (2) procedures for using the categories to make classroom observations.

The verbal interaction categories are shown in exhibit 9.6. You will note that, with the exception of category 10 (silence or confusion), all categories pertain to a specific type of verbal behavior. Any verbal statement that might be made by a teacher or student can be classified into one of the ten categories. This is true irrespective of grade level, subject area being taught, or personal characteristics of the teacher and students. Indeed, one of the major appeals of Interaction Analysis to educators is its universality. The ten categories can be applied to virtually any teaching situation. For example, a first-grade reading group and a graduate-level seminar could be compared for similarities and differences using the system.

You will note in exhibit 9.6 that the categories are classified into two kinds. Some verbal behaviors are responses a teacher might make to a student comment (categories 1, 2, and 3) or responses a student might make to a teacher comment (category 8). Other verbal behaviors are intended to initiate communication. Either a student (category 9) or the teacher (categories 5, 6, and 7) can play the role of initiator. Categories 4 and 10 are neutral. They reflect neither response nor initiation.

Another way of grouping the ten categories into larger units is to consider who is the speaker during a particular verbal interchange. In a classroom situation, the speaker is either the teacher or a student.[12] Exhibit 9.6 shows that the first seven categories are used to code teacher statements. Categories 8 and 9 are for coding student talk. Category 10 reflects confusion or the fact that no one is speaking at a particular point in time.

The most critical distinction in Flanders's system is between response and initiation. If you think about the way in which you communicate with others, you will realize that you do one of two things: (1) respond to what someone else has said by listening or by offering a comment that directly relates to the other's communication; or (2) take the initiative by putting forth an idea, by giving a direction, or perhaps by criticizing what someone else has said or done.

When a teacher makes a responsive comment (categories 1, 2, or 3), he or she is said to be using an "indirect" style of teaching. You will note that these indirect behaviors are also associated with positive affect—accepting feeling, praising, and acknowledging students' ideas. When a teacher initiates a verbal interchange (categories 5, 6, or 7) he or she is said to be using a "direct" style of teaching. According to Flanders, asking a question is neutral—neither direct nor indirect.

FLANDERS INTERACTION ANALYSIS CATEGORIES* (FIAC)

Teacher Talk	Response	1. Accepts feeling. Accepts and clarifies an attitude or the feeling tone of a student in a nonthreatening manner. Feelings may be positive or negative. Predicting and recalling feelings are included. 2. Praises or encourages. Praises or encourages students; says "um hum" or "go on"; makes jokes that release tension, but not at the expense of a student. 3. Accepts or uses ideas of students. Acknowledges student talk. Clarifies, builds on, or asks questions based on student ideas.
	Initiation	4. Asks questions. Asks questions about content or procedure, based on teacher ideas, with the intent that a student will answer. 5. Lectures. Offers facts or opinions about content or procedures; expresses his own ideas, gives *his own* explanation, or cites an authority other than a student. 6. Gives directions. Gives directions, commands, or orders with which a student is expected to comply. 7. Criticizes student or justifies authority. Makes statements intended to change student behavior from nonacceptable to acceptable patterns; arbitrarily corrects student answers; bawls someone out. Or states why the teacher is doing what he is doing; uses extreme self-reference.
Student Talk	Response	8. Student talk—response. Student talk in response to a teacher contact that structures or limits the situation. Freedom to express own ideas is limited.
	Initiation	9. Student talk—initiation. Student initiates or expresses his own ideas, either spontaneously or in response to the teacher's solicitation. Freedom to develop opinions and a line of thought; going beyond existing structure.
Silence		10. Silence or confusion. Pauses, short periods of silence, and periods of confusion in which communication cannot be understood by the observer.

*Based on Ned A. Flanders, *Analyzing Teaching Behavior,* 1970. No scale is implied by these numbers. Each number is classificatory; it designates a particular kind of communication event. To write these numbers down during observation is to enumerate, not to judge, a position on a scale.

Exhibit 9.6

Student verbal behavior is summarized in two categories. The student is either responding in a narrow way to the teacher (category 8), or the student is expressing personal ideas and opinions (category 9). It is thought that a teacher's use of an indirect style of teaching (categories 1, 2, 3) encourages students to increase the frequency with which they offer their own ideas and opinions (category 9). In contrast, a teacher's use of a directive style (categories 5, 6, 7) is thought to channel students' ideas and behavior to meet teacher expectations (category 8).

This brief glimpse into Interaction Analysis reveals that it is both simple and complex. All classroom communication is coded into ten categories, yet the data yielded by these categories can lead to complex analyses of the teacher's behavior. The intent of a teacher's communication can change from one second to another; these changes can form patterns that reveal a teacher's characteristic way of interacting with students. For example, one teacher's routine may be to ask a question (category 4), elicit a narrow student response (category 8), and respond in turn by asking a new question (category 4). This is a 4-8-4 pattern. Another teacher may be in the habit of asking a question, eliciting an open-ended student answer; then the teacher praises the student for the quality of the answer, builds on what the student has said, and initiates a new question. This is a 4-9-2-3-4 pattern.

As teachers are exposed to Interaction Analysis data on their classroom teaching, they are likely to move toward more complex and varied verbal behavior patterns. They also should become more aware of their verbal behavior and how it affects student learning.

At this point you have probably asked yourself, "Which is better —an indirect or a direct teaching style?" Research on Interaction Analysis suggests that use of an indirect teaching style is associated with more positive student attitudes and higher student achievement.[13] But this does not mean that a direct style is necessarily poor teaching. Flanders suggests that there are times in the curriculum when the teacher needs to be direct, as in presenting new content to students and in giving directions. In direct teaching, though, there is opportunity to use some indirect verbal behaviors. For example, the teacher may be giving an extended series of directions for doing an experiment (category 6). While doing this, the teacher might consider pausing to praise or encourage the students for their efforts and success in following directions (category 2).

A similar situation can occur in indirect teaching. For example, the teacher may be moderating a discussion in which students are encouraged to state their own opinions on an issue (category 9). The teacher may acknowledge students' ideas (category 3), encourage silent students to talk (category 2), and verbalize awareness of the feelings that underlie students' opinions (category 1). All these are indirect verbal behaviors. At some point in the discussion, though, the teacher may discover that students are misinformed about a particular issue and so decide to interrupt the discussion temporarily to provide information (category 5) and direct students to do homework reading (category 6). Thus, the teacher has interspersed direct teaching into a predominantly indirect, student-centered lesson.

We conclude this analysis of direct versus indirect teaching by advocating that teachers need to be *flexible,* as do supervisors (see chapter 5). They need to be able to use both direct and indirect verbal behaviors. A particular lesson may require a predominantly direct style, but the skillful teacher will find opportunity to use a few indirect behaviors as well. Another lesson may require a predominantly indirect style, but again the skillful teacher will find opportunity to interject new information and may find it necessary to direct students' ideas so that they are productive.

This is only a brief introduction to the ten categories of the Flanders Interaction Analysis System. We trust that it is enough to help you understand why these classroom observation categories have captured the attention of educators worldwide and why it has been used extensively in teacher supervision.

Timeline Coding (Technique 21)

In describing Interaction Analysis, we stated that it has two main features. The preceding section discussed the first feature, namely, the ten categories for coding verbal behaviors. The other distinguishing feature is the way in which the behaviors are coded by the observer.

Exhibit 9.7 presents several examples of timelines used in conjunction with the Flanders Interaction Analysis System.[14] The first thing to notice about a timeline is its columns. Each column represents a three-second interval. The three-second interval is long enough that the observer need not become preoccupied with recording data. In most lessons there usually are several periods of time lasting a minute or more when only one interaction category is being used. (These are usually categories 4, 5, or 6.) The observer can relax during these time intervals until the pace of interaction increases again.[15]

TIMELINES

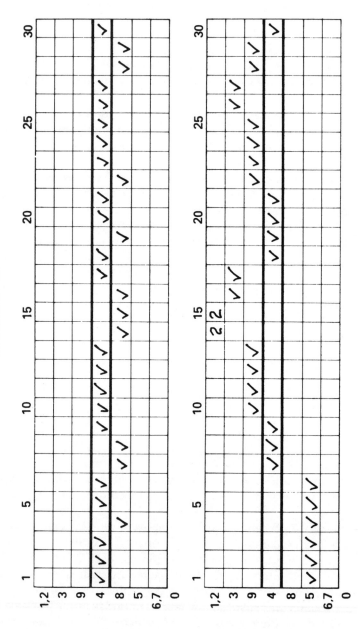

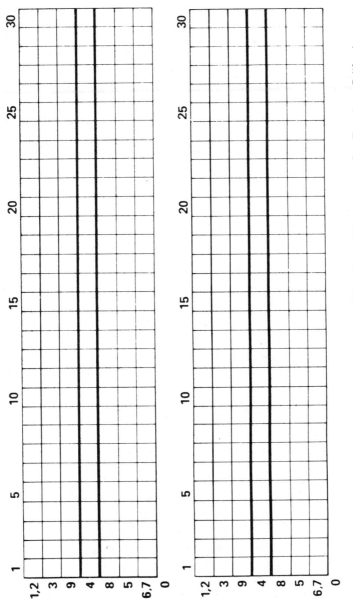

Exhibit 9.7

The timelines shown in exhibit 9.7 have thirty columns for recording thirty discrete observations. Since an observation is made every three seconds, each timeline covers about one and one half minutes of classroom interaction.

The other salient feature of an Interaction Analysis timeline is the rows. Each row represents one or two categories. The middle row is for teacher questions (category 4), which often are a stimulus for a series of interactions between teacher and students. Categories reflecting an indirect teaching style (1, 2, and 3) are above the middle row, as is the category reflecting open, student-initiated responses (category 9). Categories that indicate a direct teaching style (5, 6, and 7) are below the line, as is the category for structured, restricted student responses (category 8).

Category 10 (silence or confusion) is not represented by a discrete row. Tallies for this category are made below the timeline. Several categories (1 and 2, 6 and 7) share the same row in order to conserve space. The observer can use differentiated tallies (e.g., a check mark for category 1 and a slash for category 2) if he or she wishes to identify these categories separately on the timeline.

The organization of the Interaction Analysis categories on the timeline makes it easy for supervisor and teacher to detect verbal patterns that occurred during a lesson. For example, a majority of tallies above the middle row indicates that the lesson was indirect in style. A majority of tallies below the middle row indicates that the lesson was direct in style.

The first timeline in exhibit 9.7 is characterized by alternating 4s and 8s. This pattern suggests that the teacher was engaged in a rapid question-and-answer interchange with students, with the level of discourse probably focused on fact recall.

The second timeline in exhibit 9.7 suggests a richer, more indirect dialogue. The teacher starts by giving some information on a curriculum topic. Then students are invited to offer their own ideas on the topic. After each student response, the teacher takes care to acknowledge the student's idea and, in some cases, to praise it.

Many other interaction patterns can be revealed through timeline analysis. When teachers first become exposed to Interaction Analysis, they typically find that they use a few simple patterns in interacting with their students. As they see these patterns recorded on a timeline, they are likely to become dissatisfied and to explore how they can become more flexible in their use of verbal behavior. Sometimes, but not always, this involves a shift from a more direct to a more indirect style of teaching.

Our discussion of timelines has focused on its application to Flanders Interaction Analysis categories. Timelines are a generic recording device, however. With a bit of creativity on your part, you can imagine other behaviors that can be inserted in place of the Interaction Analysis categories (e.g., teacher feedback or teacher questions). Also, the three-second interval represented by the columns of the timeline can be varied. You may want a shorter or longer time interval depending on the observation categories included in your timeline system.

Notes

1. Many other checklists are described in Gary D. Borich and Susan K. Madden, *Evaluating Classroom Instruction: A Sourcebook of Instruments.* (Reading, MA: Addison-Wesley, 1977).
2. Student Reaction Center, Western Michigan University, Kalamazoo, MI 49001.
3. Roy C. Bryan, "The Teacher's Image Is Stubbornly Stable," *Clearing House* 40 (1966): 459–60.
4. Roy C. Bryan, "Some Observations Concerning Written Student Reactions to High School Teachers" (Kalamazoo, MI: Educator Feedback Center, Western Michigan University, 1968).
5. The Pupil Observation Survey was developed at the Research and Development Center for Teacher Education, The University of Texas.
6. Bruce W. Tuckman, "A Technique for the Assessment of Teacher Directiveness," *The Journal of Educational Research* 63 (1970): 395–400.
7. The importance of this teacher behavior is discussed in Mary B. Rowe, "Science, Silence and Sanctions," *Science and Children* 6 (1969): 11–13.
8. Ned Flanders, *Analyzing Teaching Behavior* (Reading, MA: Addison-Wesley, 1970).
9. These rating checklists are called Teaching Analysis Guides by Joyce and his colleagues. They are included in a set of three books: Marsha Weil and Bruce Joyce, *Information Processing Models of Teaching* (Englewood Cliffs, NJ: Prentice-Hall, 1978); Bruce Joyce and Marsha Weil, *Social Models of Teaching* (Englewood Cliffs, NJ: Prentice-Hall, 1978); Bruce Joyce, Marsha Weil, and Bridget Kluwin, *Personal Models of Teaching* (Englewood Cliffs, NJ: Prentice-Hall, 1978).
10. Flanders, *Analyzing Teaching Behavior.*
11. A brief, excellent package for learning how to use this observation system is *Interaction Analysis: A Mini-Course* by Ned Flanders and his colleagues. It is available from Paul S. Amidon and Associates, Inc., 4329 Nicollet Avenue South, Minneapolis, MN 55409.
12. Some classes may have a guest speaker or a teacher aide. In this situation you may wish to adapt the Flanders Interaction Analysis System to accommodate the additional speaker(s).
13. See references on page 27.
14. The use of a timeline to record Interaction Analysis data is a relatively recent development. If you learned the system some years ago, you may be familiar, instead, with the use of matrices to record and interpret Interaction Analysis data.

We present the timeline method here because we believe it is generally superior to matrices in ease of coding and interpretation.

15. When a simple interaction category occurs for any length of time, the observer may abbreviate the recordkeeping process. For example, if the teacher launches into an extended explanation of a concept, the observer may place a few tallies in the row designated by category 5, and then draw a short arrow with a note indicating approximately how many minutes or seconds this category of verbal behavior was used.

Unit Exercises

Multiple-Choice Items

Answers are on page 192.

1. Teachers' use of redirection and probing can be analyzed by:

   a. the verbal flow technique.
   b. the at-task technique.
   c. the movement pattern technique.
   , d. selective verbatim of teachers' questions.

2. Research has shown that the most common form of teacher feedback is:

   a. praise.
   b. criticism.
   , c. repetition of what the pupil said.
   d. acknowledgment and elaboration of what the pupil said.

3. The figure shown to the right is most likely from a(n):

   a. selective verbatim record
   , b. verbal flow record.
   c. at-task record.
   d. movement pattern record.

4. The figure shown to the right is most likely from a(n):

   a. selective verbatim record.
   b. verbal flow record.
   , c. at-task record.
   d. movement pattern record.

   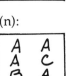

5. The specific emitters and targets of verbal behavior in classrooms can be identified most effectively by the:

   a. verbal flow technique.
   b. movement pattern technique.
   c. Student Perception of Teacher Style checklist.
   d. Flanders Interaction Analysis.

159

6. The technique most closely related to the ethnographic method in anthropology is the:

    a. video recording.
    b. timeline coding technique.
    c. anecdotal record.
    d. selective verbatim.

7. When first exposed to a videotape of their teaching behavior, teachers tend to focus on:

    a. their physical appearance.
    b. their students' physical appearance.
    c. their students' at-task behavior.
    d. verbal flow patterns.

8. The Teacher Image Questionnaire and the Pupil Observation Survey are examples of:

    a. supervisor-administered checklists.
    b. teacher-administered checklists.
    c. school-principal-administered checklists.
    d. student-administered checklists.

9. In the Flanders Interaction Analysis System the behaviors of accepting feelings, praising, and accepting ideas are examples of:

    a. teacher initiation.
    b. teacher response.
    c. student initiation.
    d. student response.

10. In timeline coding columns are used to indicate _____, and rows are used to indicate _____.

    a. teacher initiation, student response
    b. teacher response, student initiation
    c. behavior categories, time intervals
    d. time intervals, behavior categories

Problems

The following problems do not have single correct answers. Possible answers are on pages 194–95. Your answers may differ from ours yet be as good or better.

1. A teacher under your supervision has a concern about how she "comes across" to students but can't get any more specific than this in stating the concern. What observational techniques might you select? Why?

2. A teacher tells you he has several problem students in his class. The students create class disturbances and spend little time engaged in learning. The teacher would like you to collect data on their behavior that would help him better understand why these students are a "problem." What observational techniques would you consider using? Why?

3. Here is a verbal flow chart made of an actual sixth-grade class. The teacher had given a presentation on a social studies topic and, at the time of the classroom observation, she was discussing the topic with the class. What inferences and recommendations for changes in the teacher's behavior might you make based on the verbal flow data? (See page 162.)

4. The following is a transcript of the first few minutes of an actual lesson in a junior high school class. First, make a selective verbatim of the teacher's feedback statements. Second, code the transcript on a timeline using Flanders Interaction System. Assume that each line of the transcript represents a three-second interval.

(*T* = teacher, *S* = student)

T: Who knows what a population explosion means? Who knows what it means?

S: I think it means like too many people, there's too many people living in like all over the world, there is just too many people. The population has just increased, the amount of people is just going up. It's just expanding, put it that way.

T: All right. How many people are here in the world right now?

S: A couple of billion.

T: A couple of billion. Any other guesses?

S: I'd say about six million.

T: Six million.

S: There is only about a billion.

T: Only a billion.

S: I'd say about three billion.

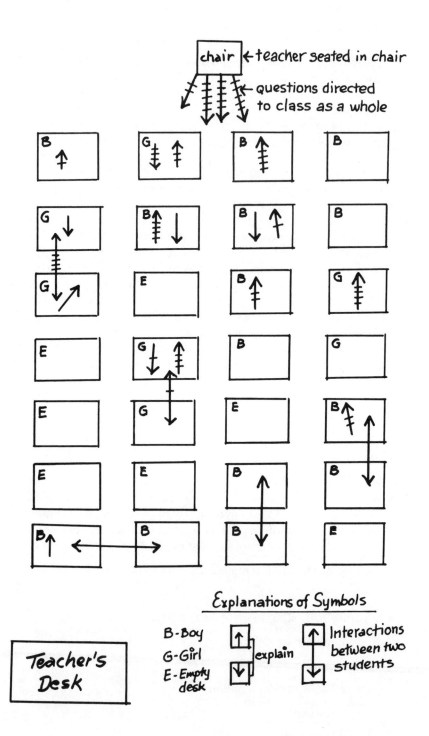

T: About three billion. All right, Mary is closest because it is over three billion people in the world today. A couple of billion, that is a billion less than three billion, though, unless you meant a couple of billion or three. All right, what do they mean by squeezing to death? What do we mean by squeezing to death, Liza?

S: Well, there will be so many people in the world that there will be no place for them to go, and they squeeze.

S: Well, it means that there are a lot of people that are just barely making it in their life. You know, they don't have much money.

T: All right, there are a lot of people that are just barely making it.

Unit IV

Case Studies and Issues

10

Studies of Clinical Supervision

A Case Study

Alan was working at his desk when he overheard his name being used. "Let's get Alan to work with her; he's acceptant." Several supervisors had gathered across the room to discuss Bernice, a beginning teacher who was not doing well in her junior high assignment and had not responded to the efforts of other supervisors. Alan wasn't sure what the supervisors meant by "acceptant," but assumed that it was similar to "open-minded," so he took the assignment and went out to meet Bernice.

His first impression was that she was shy, sensitive; he also noted that she was somewhat overweight and scared. Other supervisors had given her lots of advice, some of it contradictory; but she felt that none of it had been very helpful in solving her problem of how to deal with the young adolescents in her charge.

Alan and Bernice talked for a while. After she had a chance to describe her problem as she saw it, Alan suggested, "Why don't we have a look at how you interact with your students and see if that gives us any clues?"

Bernice agreed. She was ready to try anything. Alan suggested making a videotape the next day in the class that was bothering her the most and then meeting after school to view the tape and discuss it.

When Alan arrived the next day, he discovered that there were no electrical outlets in Bernice's classroom. He had to run an extension cord from the janitor's room for his tape recorder. Alan asked Bernice how she showed films, and she said her class had to go to a special viewing room. He could imagine some of his colleagues telling her to raise hell with the principal about getting some electric power into her classroom.

Surprisingly, the tape showed that the class was not out of control, although the students did appear to be taking some license in how they responded to their teacher. That afternoon, after Alan and Bernice had viewed the tape, Bernice commented on this fact. Alan said, "They seem to like you and are not antagonistic, but they are taking advantage of you." As they discussed the various ways that teachers deal with students, it was brought out that Bernice had not spent any time observing other teachers working with children of junior high age; hence she lacked role models with recent experience. During the next week Alan arranged for her to observe several teachers.

As Alan and Bernice worked together in the ensuing weeks, Bernice sought a teaching style consistent with her self-concept yet not so vulnerable to students taking liberties with the teacher-student relationship. She found she could exhibit more confidence and self-assurance without becoming domineering and autocratic. Alan continued to make videotapes. Afterward, he would discuss them with her as she watched and analyzed her progress. By the end of the school year she had gained enough confidence and respect so that she was offered a continuing contract to teach in that school.

Without the techniques of clinical supervision and a sympathetic supervisor, this otherwise capable teacher might not have developed the self-assurance necessary to succeed in the classroom.

A Verbatim Transcript of the Clinical Supervision Cycle

The following verbatim transcript[1] of an actual preobservation conference in a middle school has been edited only slightly. The conference was conducted by a supervisor from outside the school, not by the building administrator.

The teacher is a young woman in her second year of teaching. Her first year was not successful; rather than dismiss her, however, she was transferred to another school. The first quarter of her second year was spent in a team setting. The observations that follow were made during the first week of the second quarter, when she was back in a self-contained classroom. The lesson being observed was intended to help students generalize about why cities grew where they did.

Planning

S: What are you going to do seventh period today?

T: OK; the first thing I'll do is tell them the subject of today is "why the cities grew and where they grew." Most of the time I'll probably be at the board, and they'll give me a reason why—why they think a city would develop, either around a river or whatever. Then with the examples, I'll have them give examples, and if they're not bringing out, you know, that many examples, I'll give them a name of a city and ask why they think it would develop.

S: They'll come out with them, just about general ideas of the city?

T (*interrupts*): Yes, you know—climate, rivers, railroads, and stuff like that. Then talk about why some—well, these are the cities that grow as they think. And then talk a little bit about why some cities may have at one time been growing and whether they just kind of stopped growing or died altogether, and what could have possibly caused stuff like that.

S: The growth of, and demise of, cities. Hopefully through questions?

T: Yes, through what they think.

S: And if they don't come out with it, then you're going to say what about Chicago? Or what about Miami?

T: Yes, what could have maybe made it happen there.

S: And then what?

T: OK; then talk a little about why Los Angeles would have grown.

S: Now, are you going to lecture about this?

T: No, just ask them why. You know, have them bring out ideas. Well I think I'll just, without going into a long thing with the history of development—that's not what I wanted—but just to bring it back to L.A. You know, the water here, the climate here, and things like that; and what made people come here.

S: You think they'll know about this? They already have enough information to bring out these ideas?

T: I hope so; I'm not sure. I'm not sure because I don't know L.A. kids that well yet and how much they actually know about their city. I grew up in San Diego. OK, after that, then, depending how much time is left, there's a thing, an exercise in a book, they all have them at their desk. It shows population density. The first example is New York and they show how New York is like in the eighteen hundreds through like nineteen thirty-four, something like that. Each little map shows how it developed, and then through there, why it developed. You know, what on the map shows why people would have moved there, and then the next page after that has examples of San Francisco and Boston and other cities showing their development. It goes like that through the depression years.

S: So you can take them through a general idea of how a city grows. You're going to talk about L.A., and at this time go through some of the other cities.

T: Just one other city, you know, let them look at a map and see just kind of how it spreads and maybe how far it—how they might have developed after the maps on there.

S: OK. Now what are the kids going to be doing through all this? When you're on the general part they're going to be answering questions or what are they going to be doing?

T: And volunteering, I hope.

S: And volunteering their own ideas. Is that what they're generally going to be doing the whole period?

T: Yes, that will be it. Yes, pretty much the whole thing. They'll be working with their notebooks at the same time—things being written down.

S: They'll write down whatever you put on the board?

T: Yes, I'll put that on the board and have them put it in their notebook.

S: And they'll put it in their notebooks?

T: Yes, write down the types of ideas that we put on the board.

S: Is that one of the rules that you've established in your class—that they keep notes?

T: Yes, they know to have a notebook. I usually remind them of that.

S: OK, what problems have you been having with your seventh period?

T: Some order, I guess; *a lot of order!* It's a pretty large class. I'm having a hard time simply with the, ah, what I'm teaching in it, I think. Until I get myself completely used to planning, I'm having a hard time planning for three preparations, all different. Last year I only taught one class five times—that's a lot easier. I feel at this point I'm probably not doing too well in any of them. I hope to eventually be able to get it, you know, enough ahead that I do have something planned ahead if only for each day.

S: OK. What can I do today? In your class?

T: I was trying to decide if I should tell you to observe. I know if I tell you to observe me, it's going to make me extremely nervous, but I know if I ask you to observe like an interaction or something—

S (*interrupts, lightly*): I won't observe *you*, I'll just observe what you do.

T: Not much difference. No, 'cause no matter what you do you'll still be observing me. I guess . . . one thing you can do is write down what I do and what I say on control.

S: Yes, either about getting them quiet or whatever may arise.

T: I was going to say something else, but I don't remember what I was going to say. No, but, anyway, about control in the classes and stuff like that. It's particularly hard in there. I'm going to try and separate some people today.

S: OK; is there anything else I can watch? Are you concerned about any particular kids? What about—

T (*interrupts*): You might look at my questions because of the setup of it all using examples of other cities. I'm not having exact questions, you know. If you could keep how we do it, kind of track of, either am I asking what I want to know or—

S (*interrupts*): Well, yes, but how will I know if you're asking what you want to know? I *can* write down what you're asking.

T: Write what I say, then, so I can look at it and see if I—

S (*interrupts*): If that's what you want, OK. So I'll keep one list of the control statements you make, and I'll keep another list of the questions that you ask.

T: OK, good. You might . . . when class starts, I'm going to divide some groups. I'm going to divide two girls. And if you could kind of keep an eye on them and see if they're still as noisy.

S: OK, are you going to divide these at the beginning of class?

T: Yes, right at the beginning.

S: So I'll know who they are?

T: Yes.

S: OK, and then I can watch those two, OK?

T: Uh, and maybe see if they still . . . I mean I may notice myself, but if they still carry on as much.

S: OK, now when can we get together for our conference?

T: Well, I have a planning period at five past two. Should I come back here then?

S: OK, that's fine. Why don't you come back here then?

Note that the supervisor followed a pattern suggested in chapters 3 and 4.

1. What will the lesson be?
2. What will you be doing?
3. What will the students be doing?
4. What problems have you been having?
5. What data will be useful?

It seems clear that the teacher has two related problems: order (control) and preparation (planned activities). The two kinds of data they have agreed to collect *do* address the problems—*verbatim questions*, since the plan (what there is of it) appears to be a teacher-led discussion employing questions as the stimulus for student contributions; and *verbatim control statements*, since "order" is a concern.

Observation

The observer was able to write "verbatim" both kinds of statements. They are listed on the following pages. The control statements were of most interest to the teacher and formed the basis for the conference that followed. (Teacher and supervisor waited until a second observation had been made before holding the conference.)

Teacher Questions

1. What do you think would be some of the reasons why cities develop?
2. But would that cause them to settle there? [Unanswered.]
3. What about things like weather conditions?
4. What about—what modes of transportation did they have at this time? [S: What are we talking about?]
5. What would be some of the major cities that developed for some of these reasons? What is a city that developed around water?
6. What other city developed about water?
7. What are possibly some cities that might have developed as trade centers? Think of people moving out west.
8. OK, what happened when people. . . . What would be the importance of cities like St. Louis?
9. What cities might have developed due to railroads?
10. What would be some of the reasons why the Miami area might have developed?
11. What would possibly be some reasons why cities would die?
12. What kind of city would die of crime?
13. In connection with the economy, what is it that would effect the death of a city?
14. What about large towns? What is it about them that makes them grow?
15. Does anyone else have any other reasons for the development of cities?
16. Where did the people concentrate?
17. Where was the land where they lived? Why would the city develop there?
18. What about when they look for enemies?

19. In what period did New York have its greatest growth?
20. What could have happened that would have increased it?
21. What about people from Europe?
22. What kept it from developing from the center? How did they spread out? In what way did they develop?

Teacher Control Statements

Day 1	Day 2

3:03 Girls, please turn around.	3:03 Class, let's have an orderly discussion today. When you want to talk please raise your hand and I'll call on you.
3:05 Girls!	
3:12 Make sure you write this down in your notebook.	
3:17 OK. Most of you have finished. We will go on.	3:23 Class! Class!
3:20 Sssssh!	3:25 Let me see hands! Let me see hands!
3:20 Ssssh!	
3:21 Mac!	3:28 Mac, if you have something to say raise your hand and I'll call on you.
3:21 Well, you don't have to listen, do you? [No.] Then don't listen.	
3:23 OK. Ssssh! Class, Girls, [One of the girls asked which girls.]	3:30 Betty! Mr. Ross!
	3:32 Mac!
3:24 Girls!	3:32 Joan!
3:25 CLASS!	3:33 Class, please give this lady your attention. [A boy asks "Which lady? She's no lady."]
3:25 Would two boys please pass out the books?	
3:27 OK. Sssssh! Turn to page 465.	3:34 Mr. Ross!
	3:35 Isn't that right, Carol? Carol!
3:29 OK! Would someone please read the introduction? Sssh!	3:36 Leslie!
	3:37 Come on, class, let's get together. If you have something to say raise your hand. I won't ask you again.
3:31 Class! You girls back there in the corner.	
3:40 SSSH!	
3:41 Class! Girls! Leslie!	
3:41 CLASS! LESLIE! SSSH!	3:39 Mr. Ross, come up here please. [Mr. Ross is the name she used for one of the students.]

Conference

Teacher and observer have questions from the first day and control statements from two days. The conference goes as follows:

T: Well, I felt better the second day than the first. But how—how did I look?

S: You know I'm not going to answer that question.

T: I know.

S: You're right, though, things were better the second day. But you already know that. If it helps for me to say it, I'll say it.

T: No, no, I mean—

S: What did you learn from the first day that made the second day better?

T: Well, that was the main thing (*pause*), to separate the people. That was the seating chart thing.

S: Well, I saw some real differences in the way you were behaving the second day than the way you behaved the first day. Your situation with Leslie the second day was much improved. What did you say to Leslie the first day? Specifically to Leslie?

T: Mostly just telling her to be quiet most of the time—umm, as I remember.

S: When did you tell Leslie to be quiet the first day?

T (*after pause*): Specifically. . . . I specifically said her name at three forty-one.

S: All right, three forty-one.

T: But she's in that corner of girls (*said in a matter-of-fact manner*).

S: Only once did you talk to her the first day. How did you respond to her the second day?

T: I, um that, well, when I wanted her to move up to the front seat, and she wasn't going to, I wasn't going to give in to her, but I was going to make her get up there.

S: Were there other situations the first day other than at three forty-one when she was misbehaving?

T: Yes, most of the time.

S: Did she realize that you were disturbed with her behavior?

T (*speaking fast*): I think she does most of the time. I didn't always direct it at her, but she knows. She enjoys that kind of thing. She likes the attention she gets, and she enjoys doing it. She's not so hard to take like when she's in a group.

S: Did she change her behavior the first day?

T: No.

S: Did she change her behavior the second day?

T: Yes.

S: OK, what did you do differently?

T: I was stricter.

S: OK.

T: Well, for some reason, umm . . . I think maybe, I think because was (*fast*) doing everything in, uh—with the whole class. That kind of thing I'm not used to being like that with a large class. I was having a pretty hard time—trying to have a whole class discussion. I wasn't paying that much attention. I wasn't as particular about the noise and stuff like that. I mean it wasn't bothering me as much. I guess, 'cause I changed around, the second day things were much more directed.

S: Were you dealing with her specifically?

T: Yes. Well, even the class as a whole it was more a direct thing. First they had to get in their seats, then they had to get in groups. They had more of a thing to do the second day which I felt more comfortable with. When was it? . . . I think I had been going about fifteen minutes, and I realized I hadn't reminded them, but some were already writing it in their notebooks.

S: Yes, I caught that. But then you said "Let's do it," and they went on and did it quietly.

T: Yes, they quietly went on and did it.

S: Because in the time that they were writing in their notebooks you didn't make one comment to them. You didn't interrupt them at all.

T: Yes, I didn't have to. So it wasn't too bad. I should have had them do it in the beginning. But . . . and maybe that would have calmed them down some.

S: They had nothing to do while you were writing on the board, except watch you write on the board.

T: Some were writing the notes, but I hadn't reminded them to put it in their notebooks. But, I figured, well, let them start now.

S: What did you do with the girls, both the group that Leslie was in and the group that was in the other corner the second day when they said, "We don't want to move; give us another chance; we're going to be good." How did you deal with that?

T: Well, I just wasn't going to take their—I said no. . . .

S: But you took it the day before.

T: Yes.

S: Why?

T: Well, I remember—the first day—I don't know if I was—OK, for one thing it was the first day you were there. For another, it was the first day I had the whole class in my room. I guess I was nervous.

S: OK.

T: As I remember, I told them to be quiet, but that wasn't really bothering. And because it was so much more of an unstructured thing. So I remember I wasn't simply as much aware of it.

S: But it bothered you enough several times for you to tell them to be quiet.

T: I said it because I had to keep them down, quiet, but as far as I think I was almost at the point of "OK, you little roost of girls in the back, you can talk all you like." And subconsciously I think that—

S (interrupts): And the second day you weren't going to take that, basically?

T: Yes. And I was putting them in those seats. I said, "You know, you know you're bigger kids than that." But it didn't work with those—especially with those groups of girls, they were the main thing, the main thing in there. So they're pretty much divided up now.

S: Well, I saw a real difference between the way you behaved on the two days, the two successive days.

T: Well, I knew it. I think it was because I had more confidence than because it was more—they were just simply doing more of a particular thing. And hopefully when I did things like with the board, you know, more things with the board, I'm going to do them in short periods of time to make sure I get used to it. I—it was a little too much for me.

S: OK, I think you were doing some things for too long a period of time, and that was one thing.

T: Some of the kids, you know, getting so—it became, I think, too much; I think, the kids not being used to it, it became just a little too much for too long, and I should have started. I've done stuff at the board for other classes, but I've kept it in smaller amounts.

S: OK, you were doing something for too long a period of time, that was one thing.

T: Yes.

S: Let's see if we can summarize some things here to help make what you said more obvious. You hadn't given them instructions to do things in their notebooks which would require them to do something. You weren't dealing specifically with the people, like Leslie, who were causing the problems. What you were doing wasn't really changing their behavior. OK, that's three real differences between the two days. OK, can you think of anything else? I don't know that I can.

T: Not specifically.

S: Can you identify the five or the eight or I don't know how many kids who were the problem Tuesday? Can you think back and, not necessarily by name, but know who they are?

T: OK, Lisa and that, those are the girls on that corner. Mac becomes a problem simply because he's so anxious, for one thing. The first day I think I was more worried about you and what I was doing than worrying about the kids and that I wasn't too strict.

S: There's a fourth one. Be worried about the kids, individually rather than as a group. That's a fourth thing that's a difference in the way you were behaving Tuesday. You got to deal with the kids as kids rather than just as a class. You dealt with them individually, which is very important.

T: Yes.

S: OK, how many kids did you talk to in trying to control? How many names did you mention?

T: In the control? Hardly any.

S: That was a reflection of that attitude.

T: Yes, yes, it was.

S: So, you were dealing with them as a class rather than as individuals. It was such a difference. You were a different person in the way that you handled the situations.

T: Yes, and I knew it.

S: And they knew it. There was no doubt now in Leslie's mind that you are the teacher.

T: Yes, she just kept sitting there while I was talking.

S: You know that was—my feeling was that, that was a real significant fifteen seconds when the kids very nicely, very softly pleaded with you to give them another chance.

T: She wouldn't yell at me or anything like that.

S: No, no, not Leslie. But the first time, they just kind of, "Ah, come on." You know, they acted differently toward you. And you said, "Nope," and then followed that up five minutes later with an outright confrontation with Leslie when she said, "I will not." Any number of teachers, unsuccessful teachers, would at that moment have said, "OK." They would have said OK and just let it go at that. Let's summarize what we've discussed before we look at those questions you wanted me to record.

T: I'll summarize, but the bell is going to ring in five minutes, and I have to get to class. Let's see—I need to plan things for shorter time periods. Umm, the kids have to be busy; I should use their names and get them involved; and, let's see—you said there were four—oh yes, deal with individuals.

The conference was successful in identifying some changes that offered promise. The supervisor might have seized on the opportunity to follow up the teacher's comment about things being "more directed" the second day to emphasize the value of planned activities. It is interesting to note that the supervisor's theme throughout the discussion seems to be the importance of dealing with individuals whereas that is the last point the teacher remembers (or almost forgets) in her summary.

In analyzing the control statements, one might point out that during the first twenty minutes on day 1 there were reprimands every couple of minutes and the "lesson plan" for discussion, which was "pretty much the whole thing," was over at 3:25 when two boys were asked to pass out the books (which she said would be "at their desks"). During the second day there were twenty minutes of uninterrupted time from 3:03 to 3:23. The teacher could be given specific praise for this improvement.

Some supervisors might go beyond the point that was made about dealing with individuals being better than dealing with groups and add that, when possible, dealing with individuals in private (or at least at their seats rather than in front of the whole class) is even better. Many other aspects of the lesson could have been chosen to discuss. Other uses could have been made of the data. More emphasis could have been placed on the actual data and less on the teacher's recall.

Nevertheless, the teacher gained enough from this and subsequent observation, analysis, and practice to improve her teaching and hold her job.

Notes

1. John Hansen, *Trainer's Manual*, to accompany Keith A. Acheson and John H. Hansen, *Classroom Observations and Conferences with Teachers* (Burlingame, CA: Association of California School Administrators, 1973). Used by permission of T.I.P.S., P.O. Box 20011, Tallahassee, Florida 32304.

11

Questions About Clinical Supervision

Our aim throughout this book has been to describe the techniques of clinical supervision in a clear, straightforward manner. Yet, we know that educators need to challenge the rationale, procedures, and implications of clinical supervision before they can accept it. They must "try it on for size" before they decide whether to adopt clinical techniques as part of their supervisory style.

This chapter helps you through this process by presenting issues and questions frequently raised in courses or workshops about clinical supervision. The various issues and questions are organized around conflicts between teacher and supervisor, problems in conferences and observations, finding time for supervision, and the supervisor's role.

Conflicts Between Teacher and Supervisor

What should the supervisor do when supervisor and teacher have a disagreement?

Even in good supervisory relationships, teacher and supervisor occasionally find themselves in disagreement. They may disagree about such instructional matters as the appropriateness of role playing for a particular lesson, the use of behavioral objectives in instruction, or the desirability of verbal praise following a correct answer by a student. Disagreements occasionally touch on deeply held values—for example, the teacher's style of dress or the amount of freedom to allow students in the classroom.

The supervisor may decide to avoid overt disagreement by withholding his own values, beliefs, and preferences when they conflict with those expressed by the teacher. At the other extreme the supervisor may decide to advocate his own views at the expense of the teacher's. A supervisor at this extreme might say, "I know you don't mind if students talk quietly to one other when they've finished their assignment, but *I* think you should make them stay in their seats and start another project."

In some situations the supervisor's only sensible course of action is to confront the teacher. This is true when rules and regulations of the school, school district, or other legitimate authority are involved. Suppose the school district has a policy that elementary grade children will receive at least thirty minutes a day of science instruction. If a teacher tells the supervisor, "I don't cover science in my class because there are so many other subjects that are more important for young children," the supervisor has a responsibility to inform the teacher of school district policy.

A supervisor who overtly disagrees with a teacher should explain in depth *why* he disagrees. In the above example, the supervisor might explain why the school district adopted their policy concerning science instruction. The teacher still may disagree with the policy, but he will be less likely to feel that the principal or school district administrators are arbitrary or authoritarian.

How can teacher and supervisor resolve their disagreements?

It depends on the nature of the disagreement. As we indicated, some disagreements can be resolved by informing the teacher about a rule or regulation that applies to the situation and the reason why the rule is needed. Other disagreements arise because the teacher is departing from generally accepted educational practice. For example, a teacher may insist that there is no point in writing comments on assignments because students don't bother to read comments. In response the supervisor may appeal to the fact that written feedback is generally considered good teaching practice. This assertion can be backed up by referring the teacher to the literature on the use of written feedback in grading students' papers.

If a teacher remains unconvinced after discussion of a disagreement, the supervisor must consider whether the issue is worth pursuing further. With a minor disagreement, the supervisor may wish to drop the matter rather than jeopardize the supervisory relationship.

Another approach is to make the issue the subject of a staff meeting or student-teacher seminar. Of course, any issue so treated should be depersonalized so that the teacher is not put on the spot. Discussion involving one's peers is often effective in changing opinions. The supervisor should remain open to the possibility that his views, too, may change after discussion.

We have dealt thus far with "academic" disagreements that can be resolved by rational discussion. Occasionally, teacher and supervisor are in conflict for personal reasons. For example, a teacher may not care about neatness in her classroom, whereas the supervisor places neatness next to godliness on his list of priorities. Or a teacher may feel it desirable to push students to do their best work, whereas the supervisor feels it's best for students to work at their own pace.

Teacher and supervisor in this kind of situation may simply agree to disagree about certain aspects of teaching. They still may be able to work together effectively on other aspects of the teacher's classroom instruction.

Finally, there is the case of a teacher and a supervisor who are at such loggerheads that the clinical supervision process is hopelessly thwarted. If this problem occurs in student teaching, the solution may involve assigning another supervisor to the teacher. This solution is not so easy to implement in inservice supervision. If the school principal is responsible for supervising teachers in his school, it is not so easy to assign the teacher to a school with a different principal or assign a different principal to the teacher's school. Perhaps another person in the school—for example, a vice-principal—may be able to assume supervisory responsibility. If the school district has itinerant supervisors, one of them may be assigned to work with the teacher.

Should a supervisor try to change a teacher's style?

Most supervisors have an urge to mold beginning teachers in their own image. This can be unwise if not downright impossible. The world may not be ready for another you, or the young teacher may not have the attributes necessary to do it your way. Supervisors need to keep in mind that there are usually several acceptable ways of reaching the same objective. Empathic supervisors can work effectively with teachers who exhibit a variety of teaching styles. They can help a teacher improve in ways compatible with the teacher's basic, natural style.

Should teachers and supervisors be matched according to personality type?

Few schools or colleges have the flexibility of staff necessary to make supervisory assignments on the basis of personality variables.

Also, we are not aware of any research evidence on the effectiveness of matching procedures. When there is flexibility of staff, however, the coordinator is probably well advised to take into account the characteristics of teachers and supervisors in making assignments. In preservice programs, an accepted practice is to assign experienced, mature supervisors to work with student teachers who have had difficulty in earlier teaching practicums or who are assigned to a difficult classroom. Inexperienced supervisors are assigned to work with "easy" student teachers. This matching appeals to common sense and is likely to be helpful to both teacher and supervisor.

Problems in Supervisory Conferences and Observations

What can supervisors do to help teachers who are highly defensive?

Probably most teachers are defensive about being observed, even though they may claim not to be. If the observation is perceived as being for the purpose of evaluation, it is all the more likely to elicit defensive reactions.

Many techniques advocated in this book are designed to reduce the natural defensiveness teachers experience when they are supervised. For example, defensiveness is usually lessened if the supervisor listens, uses direct advice judiciously, builds trust, and employs specific praise for observed growth by the teacher. Some teachers, however, have an extreme tendency to respond defensively even to the most tactful and skillful moves of the supervisor. Like people who panic at the thought of having their photograph taken, these teachers seem to suffer from an exaggerated self-consciousness.

A number of modifications in the clinical supervision process can be made to help deal with these special cases. One alternative is to encourage the teacher to collect his own data—for example, making his own audiotapes or videotapes. In some cases we have assured teachers that they can erase the tape if they wish, without the supervisor seeing or hearing it. Another reassuring device that has been effective is to let teachers bring a friend (or spouse) to view a videotape. A school district lawyer we know recommends permitting an attorney or teacher association representative to accompany a teacher to a conference if there is some doubt about whether the teacher will be retained.

A standard technique for helping the defensive teacher is to initiate supervision with concerns that the teacher expresses rather than with an agenda that comes from the supervisor. A skillful supervisor can take the expressed reluctance of the teacher and use it as an expression of concern. For example, the supervisor might ask, "What sorts of worries do you have about being observed?" Another approach that some supervisors have used successfully is to make it clear that the supervision-evaluation process is a joint responsibility mandated by the school district or state certification board.

Can a teacher change deep-seated traits as the result of clinical supervision?

We tend to regard several personality traits as inherent or ingrained—for example, empathy, warmth, directness, excitability. We doubt that supervisors can effect basic character changes, such as making an insensitive person into a sensitive one. Nevertheless, all these traits have observable aspects that can be developed or reduced by teachers through the use of systematic feedback. For example, an empathic person will probably maintain eye contact, acknowledge another's comments, and listen without frowning. All teachers, we believe, can learn these behaviors even though they may not reach the state Carl Rogers calls "unconditional positive regard" for the other person.

Most teachers, when presented with observational data on their behavior, are able to modify their behavior in keeping with what they recognize as more effective teaching practice. The supervisor needs skill in helping the teacher translate the symptoms of these deep-seated traits into observable behaviors that can be modified.

How should the supervisor respond to direct questions from the teacher?

In an ideal world, supervisors would provide teachers with relevant data, help them analyze and interpret the data and then the teachers would arrive at their own insights about needed changes in their behavior. The real world of clinical supervision often differs from the ideal; teachers sometimes fail to discover what the observer hopes they will notice, or the conclusions teachers reach are different from those expected by the supervisor.

A fairly common occurrence that upsets the self-discovery process is a direct question from the teacher, such as, "What do you think?" or "How did I do?" There are several ways that a supervisor can respond to such questions without placing the teacher in a dependency relationship.

One response is to return attention to the data with a remark like "Let's see" or "Let me show you some things I found interesting." For the teacher who seems insistent on getting a verbal report card before the data are interpreted, an answer like this may be appropriate: "I think we can find some strengths and also some areas for improvement. That's why we collected the data, and that's why we need to analyze it and interpret it before jumping to any conclusions."

Should a supervisor be more free to give advice to a student teacher or a beginning teacher than to an experienced teacher?

Our experience indicates that beginners are much more willing to accept advice than are experienced teachers. After a person has taught for a few years, there is a considerable ego stake involved; supervisors need to be sensitive to this fact. Advice about a specific instructional behavior can be interpreted as criticism of general teaching ability by some sensitive teachers.

Advice can be given subtly and sensitively. For example, the doctor who tells the new father, "Some fathers worry about the color of their baby's hands, until they realize that it takes a while for the circulation to reach the extremities," is doing a more sensitive job than the one who says, "Don't worry about the odd color. If you knew anything about how circulation works, you'd know that it's normal."

Isn't an observer in a classroom likely to be obtrusive?

We know people who would find it difficult to be unobtrusive in any gathering. They seem to require attention from others, or they are the sort that would stand out in any crowd. We know others who can enter a classroom, fit into the scene, and be virtually unnoticed by the class. This seems to require subordinating one's ego needs to the task at hand. Even wheeling in television recorders can be accomplished with very little distraction.

One procedure we find effective is for the teacher to announce the observer's arrival: "Mr. Jones is here to collect some information that will help me do a better job teaching." This is an honest statement that usually satisfies most students' curiosity about the observer. As the lesson proceeds, the class gradually forgets that an observer is present.

If the observer sits close to a student, the student may attempt to engage the observer in conversation. Sitting some distance from students avoids this problem.

Is there ever a time when the supervisor should interfere with the lesson being observed?

If you see a student about to harm himself or another person, you obviously should intervene. On the other hand, if a student makes a grammatical error that the teacher overlooks, it would be inappropriate for the observer to interject a correction. Younger students often come to an observer for help with schoolwork or to show something they have done. A pleasant recognition without heavy involvement is appropriate.

We sometimes notice teacher errors as they write on the chalkboard or explain lesson content. It is advisable to wait until after the class to bring these errors to the teacher's attention. To do so at the time undermines the teacher's status.

When students misbehave, many observers have a desire to intervene (especially if the observer is the building principal). Our general advice is to remain as unobtrusive as possible and interrupt only when absolutely necessary. The observer's intervention may solve the behavior problem temporarily, but it probably will not help the teacher develop techniques for dealing effectively with the problem if it recurs.

Is it possible to have too much observation data?

When we are learning something difficult, we need to concentrate on a few things at a time. Most of us have had the experience of an overzealous instructor (e.g., a friend who, in teaching us golf, overloads our circuits with admonitions about "head down, eyes on ball, arm straight, rotate hips, follow through," etc.).

Teaching is a difficult, complex process that can be digested more easily in bite-sized chunks. We have seen beginning teachers supplied with so many sources of information about their teaching that they simply did not know where to start. It is best for teachers and supervisors to single out a few key targets for change each year. They should select observation instruments that focus exclusively on the areas of desired change.

Does clinical supervision distinguish between analyzing "content" and "method" of instruction?

Let's begin our thinking about content versus method with a few illustrations. If you were working with an English teacher who employed impressive teaching methods but had spent three solid weeks on the semicolon, you'd want to discuss content, wouldn't you? On the other hand, a mathematics teacher who knows his or her subject well but is having difficulty communicating with students may profit more from work on teaching method than on curriculum.

In this book we have not attempted to describe supervisory techniques that are content specific, though it is obvious that there are differences between observing the high school band director and the primary reading teacher. Physical education, art, and foreign language teachers sometimes feel their subject matter is so special that the usual techniques do not apply. This is not the case. Observation systems may need to be adapted for specialized content areas, but the basic principles remain the same.

Can a supervisor who is not an expert in a content area help a teacher who needs supervision in that area?

There are many generic teaching behaviors, such as asking higher cognitive questions and praising students' efforts. These behaviors are generic because they are independent of the content being taught. Generic teaching behaviors usually can be observed, recorded, and analyzed by a supervisor irrespective of his expertise about the subject matter.

Other aspects of instruction are subject-matter specific—for example, pronunciation of foreign words, methods of deriving mathematical formulas, and diagnostic techniques for working with handicapped children. A teacher who needs help in these aspects of instruction is best helped by a supervisor who has expertise in the subject area. Such specialists are available in larger school districts. In smaller districts, teachers can seek help from colleagues who are knowledgable about the areas of instruction that concern them.

Can an incompetent supervisor help an incompetent teacher?

If the supervisor is totally incompetent, probably not. Fortunately, few of us are totally incompetent. Therefore the question becomes "Can you help a teacher develop a competency you do not have yourself?" To this we answer "yes." If the supervisor can recognize the observable elements of a teaching skill and can provide the teacher with relevant feedback, then improvement is likely. For example, many track coaches who cannot run a four-minute mile have helped athletes accomplish this feat.

There are limits to this ability to help in areas where we are not competent. For example, aspects of a teacher's content area may be beyond the supervisor's knowledge and understanding. Nevertheless, our experience suggests that content-area problems are seldom major concerns for teachers. Their major concerns tend to center on the process of teaching.

Most supervisors can develop the supervision skills described in this book. If supervisors will use these skills, they can help most teachers develop competence.

Finding Time for Supervision

How much time should school principals devote to clinical supervision?

We have asked hundreds of school administrators how much of their time they *ought* to spend working with teachers and how much time they *do* spend. The answers vary, but "ought" averages more than 50 percent whereas "do" averages less than 20 percent (and that, we suspect, is generous). Robert Heichberger and James Young conducted a survey of elementary teachers and found that a majority of them believed that a building principal should spend at least 35 percent of his time in supervision.[1]

If all supervisors spent 20 percent of their time on the activities described in this book we believe the quality of teaching would rise significantly. It would require one day a week (say two mornings) on the part of principals or vice-principals. They would need to schedule time for supervision, just as time is scheduled for administrative meetings or anything else high on the priority list.

Can't you learn everything you want to know about a teacher just by stopping outside his or her door once in a while?

If all the supervisor wants to know is whether the teacher is "getting by," then listening at the door periodically may be enough. Unfortunately, that seems to be as much interest as some supervisors *do* have in their teachers. The consequence is often a teacher who feels that no one really cares what happens as long as nothing gets broken.

To accomplish the kinds of improvement possible from systematic observation and feedback, time on the part of the supervisor is required.

Is there any way to compress the supervisory cycle?

Some supervisors limit the length of each phase of the clinical supervision cycle (planning conference, observation, and feedback conference) to twenty minutes. The total cycle, then, requires an hour. Another possibility is to limit the cycle to an hour but emphasize one or two of the phases—for example, ten minutes for planning, thirty minutes for observation, and twenty minutes for feedback.

A good time-saver is to use data from sources that do not require the supervisor's time as an observer. Audio recordings made by the teacher, student questionnaires, and charts and notes made by a teacher aide or colleague are examples of such data.

Another way to save time is to give the teacher a copy of the raw data to analyze before the feedback conference. For example, if the teacher has reviewed an audio recording of the observed lesson beforehand, the feedback conference can be shortened because the teacher will not need to study the data before interpreting it.

If teachers are already familiar with observation techniques such as at task and selective verbatim, the supervisor can save time by not having to explain them in the planning conference. The supervisor can present these techniques to a group of teachers at the same time, perhaps as part of the agenda of a staff meeting or preservice seminar.

What are the cost-benefits of an effective supervision program?

Recently a superintendent in a medium-sized midwestern school district told us it was going to cost about $10,000 to fire a probationary teacher in midyear because of poor teaching performance. This amount was equal to the inservice budget for all "professional growth" in that district for the year. If $2000 worth of supervisory time could have avoided this cost, it certainly would have been viewed as beneficial.

Let's consider the question another way. If a principal whose annual salary is $20,000 spends 20 percent of his time doing supervision, that is equivalent to an investment of $4000. The principal might well be able to complete six to eight supervisory cycles (plan-observe-feedback) with each of thirty to forty teachers in that amount of time. If this expenditure of time saved one firing or twenty phone calls from irate parents or fifty kids sent to the office, the principal probably would feel that supervision was cost effective.

The Supervisor's Role

Many school district supervisors place much more emphasis on evaluating teachers than they do on promoting teachers' professional development. Why is this?

One reason is that district supervisors have lacked confidence in their ability to design and conduct activities for teacher growth. Supervision as a form of professional development activity has not been a rewarding task for many supervisors. They do not feel their efforts are particularly appreciated by teachers. Research on teachers' perceptions of supervision (discussed in chapter 1) substantiates supervisors' feelings of not being appreciated. Our hope is that *clinical* supervision will reverse this condition so that teachers and supervisors both feel appreciated.

Another kind of professional development occurs through inservice education activities. Unfortunately, teachers often feel that these activities are not designed to meet their needs but to meet the needs of someone else—central office administrators, the school principal, university professors.

Clinical supervision might provide a better basis for identifying inservice needs. For example, if half the school faculty in their fall planning conference list "individualizing instruction" as a prime goal for the year, the principal can investigate the possibility of bringing resources to these teachers in the form of consultants, training, or materials.

An impediment to the identification of true needs for professional development has been the reluctance of teachers to admit that they have any problems that they cannot handle. This is partly the result of district evaluation systems. Teachers tend to receive negative evaluations for admitting problems. A better procedure would be to commend teachers when they acknowledge a problem and then, through supervision or some other method, proceed to solve it.

What can supervisors do to improve their performance?

If the techniques of clinical supervision are useful for teachers, there is no reason why they shouldn't be equally useful when applied to supervisors' performance. Supervisors should hold periodic seminars to discuss case studies and problems. With the teacher's permission, a supervisor might record a supervisory conference and play it back in the seminar so that colleagues can provide feedback on the supervisor's behavior.

Similarly, supervisors can bring observational data they collected to the seminar for discussion and feedback.

Another idea for sharpening supervisory skills is to sponsor or attend workshops on such topics as interviewing, interpersonal communication, observation strategies, and group process. Also, supervisors should continue reading about *teaching effectiveness*; as we discussed in chapter 2, this is the major goal of clinical supervision. New research on teaching effectiveness is constantly being done. Supervisors need to study this research in order to refine their ideas about what it means to be an effective teacher.

What are positive strokes for the supervisor?

Some supervisors obtain satisfaction from the status and power inherent in a supervisory role. To them the label "supervisor" connotes "superior." This self-satisfaction is not the best incentive for doing good supervision. The satisfactions that come from viewing oneself as "helpful" are much more likely to lead a supervisor to accomplish growth on the part of the teachers with whom we work.

When a teacher remarks, "Thanks for your help," the supervisor should feel rewarded for his efforts. But teachers don't always thank us. Then we need to look for intrinsic rewards such as satisfaction with the growth we see the teacher making or delight in the excellent data we have gathered to share with the teacher.

Can teachers supervise one another?

If the goal of supervision is instructional development, peer supervision can be very effective. Teachers can observe one another, provide useful feedback, and generally encourage instructional improvement. Training in clinical supervision facilitates this process. We have been pleased by teachers' response when we have offered inservice courses with such titles as "Peer Supervision" and "Collegial Observation."

One school district assigned two teachers on a half-time basis to make observations in response to teachers' requests. It was official policy that observational data would be shared only with the teacher and that the observers would not discuss the teacher's classroom instruction with anyone else. The program was well received with the observers being fully scheduled, often several weeks in advance. A budget crisis ended the program.

If a purpose of supervision is to evaluate the teacher, we doubt that peer supervision will work. This is especially true if the supervisor's evaluation will be used to make tenure or retention decisions or to award merit pay increases. Such evaluative decisions are generally viewed as the responsibility of administrators. Most teachers are disinclined to view their peers as both colleagues and administrators.

Notes

1. Robert L. Heichberger and James M. Young, Jr., "Teacher Perceptions of Supervision and Evaluation," *Phi Delta Kappan* 57 (1975): 210.

Answers to Multiple-Choice Questions

UNIT ONE

1c, 2d, 3a, 4b, 5a, 6c, 7d, 8d.

UNIT TWO

1e; 2d; 3c, e; 4e; 5c, d; 6a, e; 7d; 8c, e.

UNIT THREE

1d, 2c, 3b, 4c, 5a, 6c, 7a, 8d, 9b, 10d.

Answers to Problems

UNIT ONE

1. The supervisor might begin by acknowledging the teacher's distress (technique 27), then ask the teacher to clarify why she is distressed (technique 28). If the teacher states that she feels her teaching is inadequate, the supervisor might initiate a clinical supervision cycle in which observation data are collected to help the teacher objectively analyze her teaching. If the teacher's distress is caused by personal problems, the supervisor might assume a counselor role (see pages 14, 78) or refer the teacher to an expert source of help.
2. The supervisor might enlarge on the question by discussing all supervisory roles with the student teacher. If the supervisor's roles are both to evaluate the student teacher's performance and to help the student improve in skill, the supervisor might discuss both roles and how they relate to each other (see pages 15–17). A supervisor who has an evaluative role might allay some of the student teacher's concerns by sharing the criteria that will be used to evaluate the student teacher's effectiveness (see pages 26–33).
3. It may well be true that, *to an extent*, good teachers are born, not made. Nevertheless, there is strong evidence that a teacher's classroom performance can be improved, *to an extent*, through training (see pages 68, 184). Also, it may be true that certain aspects of effective teaching will always elude technical analysis.

But most educators (including critics of analytic methods) can identify *some* teaching techniques that differentiate effective and ineffective teachers. In other words, a possible problem with both claims is that they are too extreme.

UNIT TWO

1.*a.* Alternatives will vary. Individual conferences with students are usually better than public rebukes. Attention to planning productive activities to replace negative behavior is advisable. Reinforcing positive behavior is a powerful tool. There are many other reasonable suggestions.

  b. "If I were you, here's what I would try" is not a good opener. "Here are several possibilities; can you suggest others?" is better.

2. Responses will vary depending on the nature of the strategy chosen. Have you considered photographs, checklists, student feedback (questionnaires, reports, evaluations), getting assistance from student teachers, aides, or others?

3. The following examples for student behavior are from Spaulding. The examples for teacher conference behavior are from our own experience; the list can easily be expanded.

   Aggressive Behavior—direct verbal or physical attack, grabbing, destroying:
   "Give me that!"
   "Get out of my room!"

   Negative (Inappropriate) Attention-Getting Behavior—annoying, bothering, belittling, criticizing:
   "You don't know how to jump rope."
   "You've never had to teach a class like this one."

   Manipulating and Directing Others:
   "Tell Cynthia to get out of the wagon."
   "You ought to spend your time on kids, not teachers."

   Resisting Authority (or Delaying):
   "No, I won't do it!"
   "Would you mind repeating the question?"

   Self-Directed Activity:
   "I think I'll make a pie."
   "I'd like to make some tape recordings on my own."

   Paying Rapt Attention:
   Listening attentively as teacher gives directions
   Watching supervisor give demonstration lesson

Sharing and Helping:
  Child eagerly takes part in activity or conversation
  Teacher suggests alternative teaching activities
Transacting:
  Mutual give-and-take is present in (child's) activities.
Seeking Help:
  "Would you help me fix this?"
  "What would *you* do?"
Following Directions (Passively and Submissively):
  Doing assigned work without enthusiasm or great interest
  Trying the supervisor's suggestion for a class activity, but with
    a lack of zest
Seeking or Responding to External Stimuli:
  Observing passively, easily diverted
  Listening impassively and attending to any interruption
Responding to Internal Stimuli:
  Daydreaming
  Gazing into the distance
Physical Withdrawal or Avoidance:
  Moving away from teacher and other children
  Missing the conference appointment

UNIT THREE

1. Techniques that focus on specific behaviors, such as selective verbatim and at task, are probably inappropriate in this situation. You might consider instead a wide-lens technique—for example, an anecdotal record or a video or audio recording. Although more restricted, Flanders Interaction Analysis also may be helpful. These techniques enable a teacher to examine his or her teaching behavior and how students react to it. In examining these records, the teacher may develop a better operational definition of what is meant by "coming across."

2. An at-task analysis would be helpful in determining the percentage of time that each of these students is engaged in learning and the percentage of time that they are off task. Off-task time can be analyzed further into several categories of behavior (e.g., daydreaming, chatting with a classmate). The supervisor might also make an anecdotal record limited to the target students and the teacher's interaction with them. Another observational technique that may be appropriate is a selective verbatim in which the

supervisor records all teacher comments directed to the problem student.

3. *Inferences*
   a. Students near the front of the room do more talking than students in the back of the room.
   b. Most of the teacher's questions are addressed to the class as a whole rather than to specific students.
   c. A higher proportion of girls than boys responded to the teacher.
   d. Several students engaged in conversations with each other while the lesson was in progress.
   e. Almost half the students (10 of 21) did not participate in the lesson.

   Recommendations
   a. Have students in the back of the room move into empty seats nearer the front of the room.
   b. The teacher should consider standing so that he has a good view of all students.
   c. If side conversations between students persist, the teacher should explain why this behavior is not desirable or perhaps should move some students to different sections of the room.
   d. Direct more questions to specific students rather than to the class as a whole.

4. *Selective verbatim of feedback statements*
   All right.
   A couple of billion.
   Six million.
   Only a billion.
   About three billion.
   All right, Mary is closest because it is over three billion people in the world today.
   All right, there are a lot of people that are just barely making it.

Timeline coding:

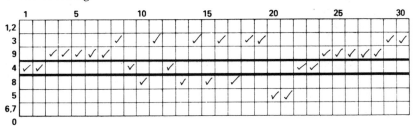

Index